bestsexwriting of the year

best sex writing of the year

volume 1

ON CONSENT, BDSM, PORN, RACE, SEX WORK AND MORE

EDITED BY **JON PRESSICK**

FOREWORD BY **BELLE KNOX**

CLEiS
PRESS

Published in the United States by Cleis Press,
an imprint of Start Midnight, LLC,
375 Hudson Street, Twelfth Floor, New York, New York 10014.

Printed in the United States.
Cover design: Scott Idleman/Blink
Cover photograph: Robin Lynne Gibson/Getty Images
Text design: Frank Wiedemann

First Edition.
10 9 8 7 6 5 4 3 2 1

Trade paper ISBN: 978-1-62778-086-5
E-book ISBN: 978-1-62778-101-5

Library of Congress Cataloging-in-Publication Data is available.

Permissions acknowledgments for the essays reprinted in this book may be found on page 224.

Molly   Hannah   Rachel   Donna   Jessie
Thank you

CONTENTS

Foreword
Belle Knox

Sex. A simple enough thing from the outside but our desires, our humanity make it so complicated. We use sex to sell everything from fast food to power tools, music to insurance; sexuality is commodified, packaged, sanitized and sold to us from every angle. It permeates every facet of our lives while remaining the most common social taboo. We use sex and the promise of intimacy to sell; however, actually selling sex or intimacy remains a hotly disputed and stigmatized topic.

In 2015, sex remains one of the most polarizing topics in the world. It's easy to forget that outside of our own, seemingly normal sex lives, the world has thousands of different stories and experiences to share that we may not otherwise have imagined. My own story is well-known enough: after being outed as a college student who moonlights as a porn performer, I was met with intense ridicule, harassment and shame. But most overwhelming was being met with curiosity. People are fascinated by sex, drawn to sex and sexuality, and perhaps the sex they are not having is the most interesting. Daring to express and expose our sexuality is not without its risks; our consequences for sharing this most intimate part of ourselves with others can be extreme. We accept pregnancy and disease as a given, but the social ramifications of what we enjoy can be severe and disturbing.

Fortunately, telling our stories can also be personally rewarding. By relaying our experiences and stories, we work towards a better understanding of ourselves. By giving up these parts of ourselves, sharing what we would normally keep secret, we become more free.

The discussions we have about sex and sexuality speak to who we are as people, from the most basic of moral concerns to our most visceral desires. In this wonderfully diverse collection you'll find pieces by Alexandria Goddard, Lynn Comella and Alok Vaid-Menon that address the wider world of sex and sexuality: who do we want to be as people and what our sex—and how we go about obtaining sex—says about us. The obligation of educators to provide people with accurate information on sex and sexuality is at the core of my beliefs, though I'm not unaware that essentially I sell fantasy, deliberately and carefully removed from context.

From Dr. Laura Agustín's passionate and thought-provoking piece on stigma and the sex industry, "Prostitution Law and the Death of Whores," to Morgan M. Page's "Crazy Trans Woman Syndrome," these incredibly diverse and personal stories strike very close to home for me. The gravitas, the pain, the outsider nature of these words wrought large on the page draws me in and speaks to me. Most of all, the authors share their deepest vulnerabilities, fears, hopes and visions with us in a demonstration of our interconnectedness as human beings.

Sexuality is extremely complex, ethereal and at times ineffable. These expressions of sexuality, however socially unacceptable we may find them, are wonderful because they expose our fantasies for consideration and the endless possibilities of pleasure and intimacy that lay beyond our narrow experiences. I hope that after reading this collection of essays, articles and narratives, your mind opens to the possibility that sexual freedom is paramount to the happiness and fulfillment of the self. Whilst reading this marvelous collection, I have gasped, laughed and at times welled with tears. We all have our stories to share and these deserve to be heard. I can only hope they give you as much as they gave me.

Belle Knox

Introduction
Jon Pressick

Sometimes I play a game. It is an easy one, and I think it is one we all enjoy—at least secretly. When I walk through neighborhoods, I wonder what is happening, right at that moment, behind the doors and curtains of a particular house. Sometimes I'll even stop and really think about it. A few of my friends will humor this game and maybe even play along. It can surely result in some laughs, but I'm serious.

I really want to know what people are getting up to. I want to know what they're doing in there. I want them to tell us.

Take a listen to Tom Waits's creepily mesmerizing track "What's He Building?" from his album *Mule Variations*. It was released around the same time that a friend and I happened upon an exhibition of photos of Australian fetishists. Both stirred my inquisitive juices. Both brought me to a world that I rarely knew of. Waits was telling me to actively wonder what was going on "in there" and the exhibition was actively telling me what was going on "in there."

Of course, it all makes me think of sex. Even if the photo exhibit had not been directly about sex, it would have made me think about sex. There is no more guarded, more secretive, more hidden subject in our society than sex. For many, sex is a conversation that just doesn't happen. Sex is the word that gets tucked under the mattress so that neither friendly visitor nor sneaky peepers will catch a glimpse of it. Sex makes us vulnerable so we hide it away as far from prying eyes as we can.

Or, at least we used to.

Sexual media has changed a lot since *Best Sex Writing* came out in 2005. At that point we were certainly intrigued and flirting with the Internet and telling stories. Remember Livejournal? But back then, if you were talking about sex on the Internet, you were predominantly talking about porn. Of course, porn is still an ever-present part of our online experiences, but out of sites like Livejournal grew an interest and passion for sex stories and sex writing.

Much is made of the Wild West nature of the Internet, it being an anything goes playground rife with the most meaningless and thoughtless content. But at the same time, it was that very abandon that allowed sex writing to become a daily fixture in our reading lives. Whether it be blogs or information sites or daily digests of sex-related news, the Internet has allowed us all to interact with sex content as often as we want—as opposed to waiting for our favorite magazines or books to cover sex topics.

Sure, magazines and books are still tremendous sources of content about the wild world of sex. But more and more, those blogs, information sites, daily digests and much more are becoming the must reads. Which is why the writers and curators of online content figure so significantly in this collection.

And while the number of outstanding sex writers and creators has exploded with the availability of our digital media, so too have the topics being highlighted. Topics that might otherwise have been considered too risqué or too bland are now freely discussed. Traditional media has always been focused on the middle of the road with the occasional foray into something like BDSM or fetish to get some attention. But the Internet has thrown open the doors of what should be talked about, from very niche and specific sexual practices to cultural critiques to the simple aspects of sex that we all missed in repressed or nonexistent sex education.

How many essays need to be written about enjoying masturbation? As many as it takes to help those who are troubled by the concept.

How many articles need to be written about which surfboard bags are best for bondage and personal confinement needs (something I remember from the photo exhibit)? As many as will fulfill that audience.

Let me tell you, there is an audience. Many different audiences, some of whom overlap and some who seek out specific content. So much sex to read about, so little time!

But that's what I'm building in here. I'm building—with the words and thoughts of so many fantastic writers—a collection of pieces that will speak to individuals, groups and cultures. Some of the topics you will read about here are very specific while others speak to all of us. Bringing them together is an attempt to throw open those doors. Pull the thoughts out from under the mattresses. Talk about sex in meaningful, thoughtful and creative ways.

After reading these works, maybe you'll open a few doors of your own.

Jon Pressick
Toronto

Captain Save-A-Ho
Fiona Helmsley

I never know what to say when I'm asked if I knew anyone who died on September 11. It's a conflict that cuts right to the strange nature of sex work—the intimate anonymity, the intimate indifference. I could be standing in front of a client's name on the Memorial Wall at Ground Zero and never know it as I never knew his last name, or have long since forgotten it.

I'm pretty sure Stephen died on Sept. 11. He worked at Cantor Fitzgerald, a company located on the 101st–105th floors of Tower 1. Six hundred fifty-eight employees, most of the people in their offices that morning, died in the attacks. I was seeing Stephen two to three times a month through the outcall escort agency I worked for in New York City, and after August of 2001, I never saw him again.

I met Stephen at a bachelor party. I hated bachelor parties. I hated them because the elements that made them such a good time for the men in attendance—the randy women, the booze, the feeling of brotherhood—conspired to bring out something very ugly in them: bravado.

The bachelor party immediately got off to a bad start. A friend of the groom called the woman who I was doing the party with—a voluptuous Latina in a platinum-blonde wig who went by the name Moët—"hefty," and she freaked out, storming off to find the friend of the groom who had set up the party, demanding an apology before she would perform. The party was held inside some kind of shipping/receiving warehouse in Manhattan and I didn't know Moët at all. I had met her just minutes before outside the warehouse, and when she stormed off, I assumed she had left me. Standing there, all by myself, in a transparent slip dress and heels, I felt like carrion for a pack of hungry wolves.

"How much for a blow job?" one man barked.

"Will you let me snort coke off your ass?" asked another.

"You and the fat one—you eat her pussy?" inquired a third.

To make matters worse, I wasn't much of a dancer. I had tried stripping once, and hated it, finding my fit in sex work that was much more one on one, much less all eyes on me. Though most of the other escorts at the agency liked doing bachelor parties because of the tips and party atmosphere, I avoided them, viewing them as frat parties for grown men. The only reason I had agreed to do this one was the soothing words of the phone girl: it was only a few guys, she'd sworn. Hastily organized. Not even a real bachelor party, more a last minute nightcap on festivities. From their voices on the phone, they sounded so drunk, she doubted they would be standing up. And Moët—bachelor parties were her forte. She was a pro.

From where I stood, Moët-less, flanked by a group of at least ten men and counting, all of whom stood upright and alert unless electing to sit in one of the circle of fold-out chairs in the middle of the room—the phone girl's assurances had been a con job, tailored to placate my insecurities. The men had probably requested a white girl for the party, and I was the only one available. Though confident I could handle the situation, I felt vulnerable and extremely uncomfortable, the primary reasons I chose to avoid bachelor parties in the first place.

"Hey! I got an idea!" a man called out from behind a large desk in a corner of the room. "Let's all play strip poker!"

"Shut up, Steve!" a sweaty man in a suit jacket whined. Most of the men were clad in subtle variations of the same ensemble, pants and suit jackets that had probably appeared much nattier earlier in the evening. "Come sit on my lap, baby, and rub those titties all over me. I know you've got some great titties under that dress," the sweaty man beckoned, crooking his finger in a come-hither motion in my direction.

"That's not fair, Ray!" the man behind the desk scolded, standing up. He looked to be about fifty, with a paunchy stomach and khaki pants worn high on his waist. He took off his suit jacket and draped it on the back of his chair dramatically, à la Demi Moore in *Striptease*. "Why should she be the only one who takes her clothes off?" he said, jiggling his big belly and unbuttoning his shirt to an imaginary beat.

"I don't know Steve, maybe because she's a *stripper*?" a voice in the group growled.

The man with the large belly opened a drawer of the desk and gestured towards me. "We have our company poker night here," he said. He reached into the desk drawer and pulled out a basket filled with unopened card decks. "You know how to play?" he asked.

I shook my head no.

"I'll show ya," he answered with a wink, handing me an unopened deck. He lowered his voice, and I leaned in closer to hear him. "It's been a *looooong* night, hon. We're just getting back from the casino, and I'm pretty sure the groom's puking in another room. Everyone here's nice, just wasted. Just do your thing, hon. These," he indicted towards the cards, "should keep the heat off of you a little bit."

"Let's play STRIP POKER!" he yelled out, rolling his belly and wiggling his hips as he threw the card decks to the men in all directions. "I can't wait to see what you're working with, Hector!"

In light of Moët's MIA status, the man's gesture made me feel like I had an ally, though one could never be sure in this business. As the men grumbled to themselves and dodged the flying card decks, I moved to the center of the chair circle, ready to start my slow, drawn-out removal of garments. There was no music, so the men's obnoxious inquiries and demands would have to serve as my soundtrack. Suddenly, Moët burst back into the room, the groom, supported by the best man, following behind her.

"Come on now, Kenny," the best man slurred. "You have to apologize to this lovely lady! Look at those lips! She could suck the chrome off a bumper!" He had lipstick on both sides of his face and wobbled on his feet. His fly was partway unzipped, and I could make out the tartan plaid of his boxer shorts through the opening.

"I never said anything to her, Mike! I swear. It was all a misunderstanding," Kenny stammered. "I was asking for a Hefty bag, for the beer cans…"

"Well, she's ready to show us all a good time, but only if you say those two magic words. Otherwise, she's out of here, and it's going to be all your fault. Right, Moët?"

Moët appeared to be in much better spirits upon reentering the room, and was wearing a man's tie around her neck, its knot perfectly aligned with the ample swell of her cleavage. Her spandex minidress looked to be at least three sizes too small and barely touched the tops of her meaty thighs. She marched over to Kenny, a slight man with feminine features and large glasses that threatened to overwhelm his face, and straddled his lap.

"Do I feel heavy to you, baby?" she purred, her large posterior extending far past his knees.

"No, baby, no! You feel just right!" Kenny exclaimed, his voice going up a few octaves as his small frame was engulfed by so much Moët.

The best man looked at me. "You gonna show us a good time, too, Courtney?"

I opened my mouth to speak, with my best feigned enthusiasm, but the man with the large belly cut me off.

"I was kind of hoping Courtney and I could be alone, Mike."

Moët gyrated deeper into the lap of the man who had insulted her. The best man surveyed the room, his eyes stopping to linger on Moët. Based on her performance, he must have decided mine wouldn't be necessary.

"All right Steve-o, she's yours, but you owe me. You can take her into that room in the back."

Another thing I didn't particularly *enjoy* about bachelor parties were these public negotiations of my services that didn't involve me.

I picked up my bag from a chair and waited for the man to lead me towards the backroom, but he just stood there, looking at me impatiently.

"What's the matter?" I asked.

"You're forgetting your cards, hon," he answered. "You want to learn, right?"

I looked over at Moët, in an attempt to communicate to her where I was going, but I couldn't get her attention. She was bent over Kenny's chair as if doing a backbend, her arms on either side of his lap, and her breasts upside down in his face. It was the one thing about the bachelor party the phone girl hadn't lied about.

Moët *was* a pro.

Stephen and I sat in the backroom for the next hour and a half playing strip poker for prudes. He didn't want me to take off anything beyond my bra and panties. All that left me to remove was my dress and shoes. He stayed in his boxer shorts.

"Thanks," I said, in acknowledgement of the diversion he'd tried to create in the other room. "But you didn't have to do that. I've done plenty of bachelor parties."

"I saw your eyes, Courtney," he said. "You looked like a deer in the headlights of life. Moët doesn't have that look." He ashed his cigarette into a plastic cup of beer. "I wouldn't have been able to live with myself. I can't get off on that. My name's Stephen, but I also have a superhero alter ego. They call me Captain Save-A-Ho."

I laughed, even though he was calling me a ho.

All of the men at the bachelor party that night, except for the groom's best man, who it was mentioned he had known since childhood, worked at Cantor Fitzgerald, in Tower 1 of the World Trade Center.

The phone girl told me that Stephen had called every night since the party to see if I was working. A few nights later, I was, and I was driven to his Brooklyn Heights brownstone. Five years before, he told me, he had split up with his wife who was living on Long Island with their teenage daughter. We went into his bedroom, and he reached into a dresser drawer and took out a small bag of white powder.

"I got this the other night at the casino. Bought it in the parking lot. I'm not really sure why," he said. "It's not my thing."

I cut a line of it on top of the table next to his bed. Its consistency was both soft and crunchy, like some kind of salt mixed with soap. I blew it behind the bed when he wasn't looking. I didn't have the heart to tell him it was fake.

We had sex and his sweat rained down on me in salty droplets. His breathing quickly became labored.

"I wish you could have seen me in my prime, Courtney," he said. "Wait," he ran into another room and came back with a photo album. There were pictures of him from high school playing football, pictures from what looked to be a college frat party, making me think of the bachelor party at the warehouse. "After your forties, hon, it's all downhill," he said. "But it was a great ride."

As I was leaving, he tipped me a hundred dollars, then made an all-too-familiar request.

"Give me your phone number, hon. We can cut the agency right out of it," he said.

I'd been down that road a million times before and had learned the hard way that unless you had some kind of special line just for them, it never paid to give a client your phone number. It ended up abused, treated like a free phone sex line or a drunken confessional. So I compromised and gave Stephen my email address, my first one ever. My mother had just bought me something she'd seen advertised on television, and had bought for herself first. Not a real computer, something called an i-Opener, similar to WebTV in that it was just the Internet, a keyboard and a screen.

Because my i-Opener had been a gift from my mom, it was registered through her account, and my email address had one very small difference from hers: the number one.

As I wrote down my email address for Stephen, I stressed the importance of remembering this digit.

"Don't forget the one," I said.

"No worries, hon," he replied.

He forgot the one, and emailed my mom.

As a sex worker, there are three questions you are asked constantly by clients. The first one is, "What's your real name?" Clients are obsessed with this question. If they can get you to tell them your real name, it makes them feel special, elevated. The relationship is still a paid one, but they now know you as anyone who is important to you in your other life does. The disclosure also negates what may be the most important veneer a sex worker has: their anonymity. It's a revelation that can be interpreted to imply "She either trusts me enough not to call out to her if I were to see her on the street, or she actually *wants* me to come up to her and say hello." The second question clients always ask is about the circumstances that led you to sex work—in their minds, the circumstances that led you astray, from good girl to bad. The third question is "What gets you off sexually?" This is usually phrased, "Now tell me what *you* like."

I had never told Stephen my real name. It was nothing against him. I had told other clients my name in the past, but because "Fiona" came across as more exotic sounding than "Courtney," in the time before the movie *Shrek* at least, to them it sounded like even *more* of a stripper name, and they never believed me. So I told Stephen that Courtney was my real name, that in spite of what he may have believed as Captain Save-A-Ho, there was nothing there to save me from—my private life and public life all blurred together as one. So when Stephen emailed my mother, he addressed the email in part to Courtney.

My mother had gotten other emails meant for me after buying me the i-Opener, but nothing related to sex work, and thankfully, Stephen hadn't written anything too revealing, just that he would like to see me again soon and had enjoyed our time together. My mother probably wouldn't have even thought the email was meant for me at all if Stephen hadn't addressed it not just to "Courtney" but to "Courtney Love." He was being funny, but I was a big fan, and my mother knew this.

In January of 2002, I was living with my mom and using her i-Opener when I came across Stephen's email, then six months old. My exit from New York City had happened hastily the previous December when I had lost my apartment in a perfect storm of Xanax addiction and unpaid rent. Clients come and go from your life, your life and theirs mixing in hour intervals and dollar allotments, and it occurred to me as I read Stephen's email that I couldn't recall seeing him after August of the previous summer.

I wrote down his email address, logged into my newly created Yahoo email account and wrote:

Stephen-
It's Courtney. Sorry I didn't get in touch sooner, but everything's just been so crazy the last few months. I can't imagine what it's been like for you. The loss of life is staggering. I don't want to say too much now, I'd rather wait for you to respond first, but I'm no longer in New York. Hopefully I'll be back soon. Just wanted to make sure you're okay and let you know I'm thinking about you.

Just as I was about to hit send, it occurred to me that my new email address might cause some confusion. It contained my real name, Fiona, followed by some numbers that were relevant to my life. I'd been so adamant to Stephen about Courtney being my real name that I figured it warranted some kind of passing explanation.

> This is my new email address. Fiona's my real name. I was just trying to keep some distance, you know?

I did make it back to New York, and in the summer of 2002, I found myself working for the same outcall escort agency I had worked for when I met Stephen. One night, my driver for the evening took me to meet a friend of his, another driver for the agency, between calls. I recognized the girl his friend was driving for the night immediately—the big breasts, the wide, shapely hips. The only thing different about her was the sable color of her wig. It was Moët.

"I remember you," she said, getting out of the car to smoke a cigarette and empty the sand from her shoes. Her driver had just picked her up from a call she had done at the beach. "We did that bachelor party together, and you ditched me."

"I didn't ditch you!" I said defensively. I had experienced the brunt end of other girls' reactions to imagined crimes in the past.

"Relax, mami," she said. "You remembered where those guys worked, didn't you? That company, in the Towers? What's your name again, mami?"

"Courtney."

"People can say whatever they want about us, and what we do, Courtney, but those men, that night, they didn't have much time left. And maybe I'm crazy for even thinking like this, but that night, I know I showed them a good time, and they went home happy. Do you know what I mean, mami? I gave them my all that night, and I feel good about that."

How a Former Porn Star's Sex Tape Helped Him Reclaim His Sex Life

Christopher Zeischegg
aka Danny Wylde

Eight years into my porn career I landed myself in the hospital after swallowing too many boner pills for work. My erection wouldn't subside, and it had to be bled out. After I started, more established performers schooled me on the pills, herbs, and injections I could use to maintain a raging hard-on for hours on end, something that was a professional requirement. A doctor told me that if I continued to take the drugs, I'd risk losing my ability to achieve an erection altogether. I was psychologically—and probably physically—dependent on ED pharmaceuticals to do my job. The choice was to either risk my sexual health or stop working altogether.

It was one of the most devastating moments of my adult life. I quit my job overnight and lost my professional identity. For the next two weeks, I followed my doctor's advice to avoid all sexual arousal. I refrained from touching myself because I had to. And because I was afraid I'd already gone too far—that I'd discover my inability to ever have sex again.

To make things even crazier, I was at the beginning of a new relationship. I'd gone on two dates with a girl and we were crushing hard. I didn't reveal the extent of my fears, but she knew we'd have to wait if we were to have sex again. And we did. The girl of two dates slept next to me during my recovery. Then she helped me to rediscover my arousal in its natural state.

Shortly thereafter, the circumstances of her life changed, leaving her with a vulnerability that matched my own. Mutual uncertainty and emotional chaos allowed us to latch on to each other in the most intense way possible. If there's something called "falling in love," our course was speed railing through it.

I looked back on my sexual history and realized that I'd done my first porn scene when I was nineteen. Prior to that, I hadn't had a serious partner. My new relationship marked the first time in my life where I could experience sexual monogamy. Sex with my girlfriend was still a form of play, but something about it became more personal. After fucking a thousand people, I felt more attached to just the one.

I didn't miss performing as much as I thought I would. But there was a part of it that I didn't want to lose completely. I liked the act of sharing my sex, and I liked the feedback. So I talked to my new girlfriend about making our own video—one that showcased the intensely personal sex we were having now.

We had to set a date or I knew it wouldn't happen.

The morning of, we had sex. And again several hours later. It was normal. We were addicted to each other's bodies. When we were alone together, I wanted as much of her as I could get.

But the day was half over and we'd done nothing to prepare for our shoot. So I began to set up a couple of tripods and attach a few lights to the ceiling. She began to apply her makeup. Not that she wouldn't have sex with me without her face made up, but this was intended for an audience. She wanted to feel beautiful.

"What if our video isn't as good as the one you made with your ex?" she asked. We were going to use the same start-up company to host our video. The content I'd created with my ex-girlfriend was a big part of its launch. However, this attempt felt different. I was still a porn star the first time I shared my personal sex. The time away from performing made me feel like a boy playing games he hadn't meant for others to see.

"Don't worry," I said. "We're perfect together. It will be."

We dawdled along. She joked about no longer wanting to do the video. I suggested that we call it off. Then she reassured me that it was still a good idea. "I want everyone to see how in love we are."

Eventually, we found ourselves in bed together. The room was bright and silent. Two cameras pointed towards us. I'd hastily set them up. They weren't even running at the same frame rate.

My girlfriend laughed. "Who makes love with the lights on?"

She was nervous, so I tried to calm her. But this wasn't a way we'd ever made love. It was usually on her bed, but she'd have music or cartoons playing in the background. We'd already be touching, or I'd look at her a certain way and it would have to happen. We might be under sheets in the morning, or getting dressed to go out at night. Never with the covers purposefully pushed aside, drowned in silence, and peering over at a pair of prosumer lenses.

The anxiety I'd felt as a young performer came back as strong as ever. We'd built this moment up to be the most perfect expression of our desire for each other. But my body was shutting down, and I was beginning to panic. I could feel the cameras on me even though nobody stood behind them.

I'd done it a thousand times with people I'd barely met, and in the most stressful environments. Yet, I couldn't get my cock hard while in bed with the girl I loved. I'd often whisper to her that I thought we could do anything together. Our post-porn video seemed like the worst act to prove me wrong.

I moved on in hopes of repairing my fractured ego, and to prove whatever it is I thought she needed to know. Her legs opened and I put my mouth on her. It should have turned me on. But I mostly thought of it as something that had to happen.

In a porn film, she'd be sucking my cock. So of course I should have gone down on her first. This video was about real life and real pleasure. I wanted my girlfriend to feel like I'd do anything to please her. Except it wasn't working. My body was dissociating from my favorite act in the world.

We tried having sex slowly, sweetly, while kissing, and lying close together. It felt like something that should be real, so I hoped that I'd be forced to believe it. Eventually, we stopped to laugh and smile awkwardly. We tried to take the pressure off ourselves. "This isn't for the video," she said. "But it's cute what we're doing."

I knelt between her legs and touched her. There was an apology inside of me that I couldn't even speak. I think she understood. She moved beyond acceptance and offered something back.

"You want to hurt me?" It was a game that had defined us from the beginning of our relationship. She saved our real-world sex video by making it real.

I didn't think of our sex as over-the-top violent, but we'd shoved needles through each other, and I'd slapped and punched her skin. Part of what made our relationship work was the constant affirmation of something slightly beyond reach. It was a mix of the utopian love seen in Disney films and the desperate, violent need to know someone written in Dennis Cooper novels. Our love had to be forever and our sex had to move beyond this life. We wanted our story to be some fucked-up fairy tale come true.

So I choked and slapped my girlfriend and made love to her on camera. She responded in a way that made me forget about everything else.

After years of porn, I thought I'd worked past the fear of performatory sex. After ending my career, I thought it didn't matter. The video with my girlfriend wasn't supposed to be a performance. It was supposed to be real.

We eventually got there—to some degree. But the reality of the first fifteen minutes (and maybe more that I edited out) is not necessarily the reality of our sex. It's our vulnerability, our attempt to share something we'd developed just for each other.

What happens thereafter is hard to define. It's different than porn and different than reality. But I like the fact that not everything is accessible. I'm teaching my body to relate in a different way, and it feels good to know that some of that is only available to my partner.

Our video shows how I make love to my girlfriend at home, but for "you." It's my nervous dip into failure because I think there's something more you want to see. With the cameras off, though, it's different. I like that you may never know how.

What Should We Call Sex Toys?
Epiphora

I use the term automatically: *sex toys*. That's what they've always been to me. As a sex toy reviewer, I spend most of my waking hours researching, photographing, testing, and writing about them. The term is commonplace, innocuous—in my seven years of blogging, I've never questioned it. Yet each day, as I wade through press releases and peruse manufacturer websites, I see that the universe seems hell-bent on introducing new alternatives into the vernacular.

While others might cry "semantics!", I think that the words we use to describe things have an impact on how they are perceived. In the case of the sex toy industry, where we have to claw and fight to even be seen as legitimate at all, this is immensely important. I do not believe that, as Shakespeare famously wrote, a sex toy by any other name would feel as good. Call something a "dong" and nobody will want to put that inside themselves.

The trend probably started with manufacturers wanting to distance themselves from the term "novelty." Understandably so: it's an old-fashioned industry word that no longer applies. It sounds trivial and frivolous. Novelties are silly, laughable trinkets from Spencer's that end up in the garbage. When I hear the word "novelty," I picture a windup vulva. Although I definitely need a windup vulva for my office, such a product is not in the same league as a $150 rechargeable silicone vibrator that comes with a sleek gift box, satin storage bag, and warranty.

Thankfully, we're also hearing less and less of the term "marital aid," with its heteronormative connotations and undercurrent of shame. But in eschewing outdated terms such as these, companies are overlooking the most basic and unambiguous replacement.

If you read my blog on a regular basis, you'll notice that I prefer to call things by their proper names. I correct and challenge coy idiots who use phrases like "C-spot" instead of clitoris, "big O" instead of orgasm, "battery-operated boyfriend" instead of vibrator, "dilly" instead of dildo, and so on. Therefore, I like the term "sex toys" because it is straightforward. It is not a euphemism. It is specific and unwavering. Sex toys are simply toys meant for play, for use during sexual activity.

At least that's what I thought. When I engaged my boyfriend in this debate, he asked whether "sex" is too narrow, whether it implies a partner. I've always considered the word to be all encompassing, but I can see his point. Still, every other option for that slot falls short.

These days it is hip and trendy for companies to come up with their own cutesy little terms—"pleasure objects," "erotic toys," "love toys"—that are clearly marketing ploys more than anything else. But this clogs the industry with superfluous terms. We could play mix-and-match all day with these words, but the bottom line is that something will always be the dominant term, and I don't particularly want that dominant term to become "pleasure products."

I'm not opposed to the idea of pleasure, obviously—and I do like the way "pleasure" refers to what a toy *does*, rather than *when* it is used. However, I feel that when we replace "sex" with "pleasure," we are sugarcoating, somehow rejecting "sex" as not representative of what we want to say. It seems like an aversion to the word "sex," which is the last thing we need. It's also less specific. "Pleasure" is much more broad, and then you tack "products" onto it and suddenly you could be referring to great music, delicious food, really comfortable couches...

The word "toy" comes with its own baggage, of course. In a certain context, it implies something childish and unimportant. You could argue that it is itself a euphemism. Yet despite these less than stellar connotations, I think it works better than "product" or "object"—words that sound sterile and generic, like jugs of all-purpose cleaner sitting on a shelf. They are not associated with anything in particular.

"Toy," on the other hand, is associated with a feeling. Not just any feeling, but a feeling that I am trying, time and again, to convey to people. Sex toys are not just mechanical devices that will get in the way of sex. They are not ominous gadgets that will turn your girlfriend into a vibrator-wielding recluse. They are *toys*, meant for adding playfulness and fun to your sex life. They inspire creativity and improvisation. In our sex-negative culture, where to enjoy sex (especially as a woman) is somehow blasphemous, this is essential.

I also believe that manufacturers invent snooty terms such as "pleasure products" as a way to artificially rise above their competition, and that's kind of shitty. Yes, LELO's products are luxurious, but are they any more sophisticated than We-Vibe's? No. It is all marketing. Besides, I can't imagine myself saying, "I have a massive pleasure product collection." Although I am picky about which sex toys I'll review, there's no need to use euphemisms when describing them.

I collect sex toys. I own over five hundred dildos, vibrators, and anal toys, which I routinely hold against my vulva (not my "lady bits"), stick in my vagina (not my "vajayjay"), press against my clitoris (not my "love button"), and push up my butt (not my "backdoor"). I don't "flick the bean"—I masturbate. Then I write about my experience in a matter-of-fact way. Because sex is normal, sex is healthy, and sex is important.

We're not helping people become comfortable with sex toys by coddling them with euphemisms. Euphemisms breed euphemisms. We all still censor ourselves when we talk about sex—a bad habit we need to break. Even in conversation, I have to bring myself to use the term "sex toys" rather than "adult" something-or-others…and I work with this stuff every day.

"Sex toys" may not be an absolutely perfect way of describing the objects I put on my genitals and in my orifices day in and day out, but it's the best option out there. By virtue of its directness, it's the most beneficial to my personal cause of normalizing these things. I believe that the less we fear offending people, the less they'll be offended. Which perhaps explains why I've been using the term "sex toys" all along—without ever thinking about it.

We Need a New Orientation to Sex
Cory Silverberg

Since the summer, I've been working on the second book in a series that offers a different approach to sexuality and gender education for young children. The first, *What Makes a Baby*, is for very
young kids, and this second one is geared more or less to kids aged
eight to ten. After many months I have a first draft, but there are
still a few topics I can't fully wrap my head around.

One of them is sexual orientation.

At first, I thought I was just struggling to figure out the best
way to explain or approach this topic for kids. But I now think my
problem is with the construction of sexual orientation itself as it's
used in sex education and research as well as in our own lives.

I've come to think that the construct of sexual orientation is
more trouble than it's worth; that what we gain from the concept
is outweighed by what we lose.

Before I explain, let me be clear that I don't think it makes sense to get rid of identities like "gay" or "lesbian," "bisexual" or "straight." For lots of people those identities are central to their experience of who they are and of the world around them. They aren't understood or lived as a choice.

I am also not arguing for some totalizing idea of sexual fluidity or gender fluidity. Some of us do have sexual desires and gender identities that are fluid, to be sure. But some of us also have strong and specific desires and identities that stay relatively fixed throughout our lives. And for others, while desire or identity may not be totally fluid all the time, they may still shift with time, experience, or opportunity.

My problem with the concept of sexual orientation is also not that it creates categories, nor even that those categories become constituted as "natural" through that magical process of forgetting that we do over long periods of time, though, truth be told, this does really bug me.

As a sex educator, I acknowledge that talking about sexual orientation can be really helpful sometimes, specifically because of those manageable categories it entails. When someone is wrapped up in knots, confused about many parts of their experience of sex, and not sure where to begin, talking about the objects of one's sexual desire and interest in terms of sexual orientation can be helpful.

But just because something works doesn't mean what we give up to make it work is worth it.

If you could forget everything you know about sexual orientation and think only of the term itself, it's not bad. I like it because it is a question that demands answers.

"Orientation" refers to one's position in space and in relation to everything around it. To orient oneself in a room is to understand one's position in relation to many other objects and people in the room, and one's relation to the structure of the room itself (the walls, the floor, the ceiling).

In this sense, what is one's orientation to sex? To sexuality?

To orient oneself in the world to sexuality would be to understand where you fit and feel in relation not only to other people and their sexuality but to sexuality as it is enacted and experienced in public: to public conversations about sex; to sex in media and culture; to sexual moments and feelings that may be impossible to put into words.

What is one's orientation to two people kissing on the street? To a sex toy store? To sexual and gender discrimination that takes the form of violence on the streets? To whatever draws our sexual interest or sparks desire?

That would be a concept of sexual orientation worthy of the human experience of sex and sexuality. It opens up a thousand questions, each question a path that will take you on a journey into your thoughts, feelings, and desires about sex.

But this isn't what sexual orientation means in sexuality research or education, or in clinical or everyday settings.

What sexual orientation refers to in practice is the position of one's sexual and romantic interests in a binary system of sex. Embedded in this idea of sexual orientation is the (false) notion that there are two sexes, and two genders, and that gender is the central focus and most important aspect of sexual desire. In other words, sexual orientation is a way of organizing and conceptualizing adult relationships that says that the most salient features of our relationships are the gender of the people we have them with.

In practice, sexual orientation poses only one question, and it is both dull and blunt: What is the gender of the people whom you are sexually attracted to and with whom you want to have intimate relationships?

This is my problem.

I came to this when I was trying to write about orientation for children. When I write, I start by just trying to get the ideas down. I don't worry about comprehension level at first; I just try to describe what I see in the world. In one of those early drafts, I wrote something like this:

Sexual orientation is the way that most adults organize their intimate and romantic relationships. Adults seem to believe that the most important aspect of who they love and who they want to be in close romantic relationships with is the gender of that other person.

So if most of the time someone who calls themselves a woman wants to be in relationships with other women, we say her orientation is homosexual. If most of the time someone who is a woman wants to be with men, we say her orientation is heterosexual. If most of the time she is open to relationships with men or women we say her orientation is bisexual.

And as soon as I wrote that and read it, I knew I had other problems. One is that neither I nor many others fit into the "man" or "woman" boxes easily. An even bigger problem is this:

Why do we need to organize our relationships based on the gender of the people we are most attracted to? Why does gender need to be the most salient aspect of the object of our desire?

If this seems like a ridiculous question to you, you don't spend enough time with kids. It's not a ridiculous question, and it's one that many kids will ask, if they feel safe enough and empowered enough to do so. It's a reasonable question, and the truth is that I don't have a good enough answer.

Instead of a good answer, when I was first asked this question, I was left with an intense feeling of "d'oh!"

Why, in the face of all the amazing ways we might describe and understand our relationships of love and lust, would we use such a narrow frame of reference? More than any other subject, it was with this topic that I felt the weight of adult sexual socialization come down on a child's understanding and experience of sexuality like a cage. Like a trap.

I was also left wondering about what sort of alternative could be offered. The alternative can't be some frameless "everyone just *is*" answer.

I think the alternative might be found in a more expansive and creative use of the idea of orientation, one that highlights our relationships to people and ideas around us, as well as our relationship to structures of power that limit our options based on things like race, class, gender, our bodies, and whom we love and lust after.

For now my tactic is to stall a bit. As I'm getting deeper into the writing, I am finding myself wanting more and more to postpone the introduction of concepts of adult sexual socialization. The cage has to come down at some point, but part of me wants to let those of us who still can roam free keep roaming just a little while longer.

I Am the Blogger Who Allegedly "Complicated" the Steubenville Gang Rape Case—And I Wouldn't Change a Thing
Alexandria Goddard

I stayed up all night screen-grabbing tweets that joked about raping and urinating on a girl they thought might be dead. Welcome to Steubenville.

The Steubenville rape case has come to an end and the verdict has been heard.

Two Ohio high school football players were found guilty of raping a drunk sixteen-year-old girl.

On Sunday, Judge Thomas Lipps ruled that Trent Mays, seventeen, and Ma'Lik Richmond, sixteen, digitally penetrated the West Virginia teenager known only as "Jane Doe."

Their punishment? Richmond will be held at a juvenile detention facility for at least a year and Mays for at least two years. Both are required to register as juvenile sex offenders, and the juvenile system can hold them until they are twenty-one years old.

As a blogger who first reported on the Twitter messages surrounding the alcohol-fueled party—many messages later deleted—it is sometimes surreal to look back and revisit the events of the past eight months.

When I first wrote about the unbelievable events that took place in this town where I lived for five years—events which culminated in a passed-out female minor, Jane Doe, being carried around unconscious as men from the high school football team boasted about rape on video, tweeted jokes about violating her and, at one point, disgustingly said how "some people deserve" to be urinated on, I had NO clue the firestorm that it would cause.

All I wanted was justice for Jane Doe. And now with the verdict in, I am proud to have played any small part in that. And I'm proud of the thousands of people—from Anonymous to Roseanne—who rallied to this young woman's defense, even though no one seemed to do so the night that it mattered.

The night she will never get back. The night of her rape.

I lived in Steubenville for about half a decade. Over the years since I have moved away, I kept in touch with friends and would occasionally read the local websites to see what was happening back in my old hometown.

On August 22, 2012, I learned of the arrest of two Steubenville High School football athletes for rape, kidnapping and material containing a nude minor. I would later learn through my online research that the teens had been to a series of end-of-summer parties and the victim was sexually assaulted at a third location.

Today as I read the sickening text messages from the trial—from men who are not even on trial themselves, I found myself sobbing once again. "How dead is she?" "I wanna see the vid of u hitting her with your weiner." "She looks dead lmao."

Disgusting.

Initially, the media did not present a lot of information about this case and that struck me as odd because I knew from having lived in Steubenville that this was going to be a big deal.

I did a few Google searches and wasn't able to come up with much so I went to the high school football website and made a list of names. I read a few local high school forums to get a gist of who was who and then started searching Twitter. I figured I'd see what the other kids were saying about the case. You can learn a lot through these conversations.

Through researching, I was able to determine the boys' names and found their accounts on Twitter. The accounts were unprotected, and I started clicking through Twitter conversations. I was amazed at how much information I was able to obtain with the first two hours of searching. I had a decent idea by that time of what parties they were at, some of the names of those in attendance and knew that a photograph had been circulated.

I actually stayed up all night reading Twitter accounts. By the time I reached partygoer Michael Nodianos's Twitter account, I was horrified.

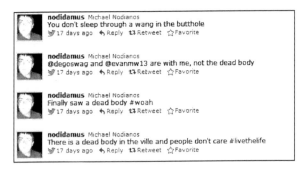

nodidamus Michael Nodianos
I don't want to leave her now, you know I believe and how #Something
17 days ago ↰ Reply ↳ Retweet ☆ Favorite ⚬2

nodidamus Michael Nodianos
Some people deserve to be peed on #whoareyou
17 days ago ↰ Reply ↳ Retweet ☆ Favorite ⚬6

Twitter screengrab via prinniefied.com

I could not believe some of the things this young man was saying about this young girl. Things like "some people deserve to be peed on #whoareyou" and "you don't sleep through a wang in the butthole." I also knew that there was a 12:29-minute-long video as I had found a copy of the thumbnail on Google cache, and was mortified that it had been tagged with words such as "drunk," "rape" and "offensive."

I just remember thinking to myself—who raised these kids and why aren't more kids arrested? And the ultimate question: If so many kids were tweeting about this rape, WHY DIDN'T ANYONE DO ANYTHING? TO STOP IT?

As I got deeper into the Twitter "evidence"—because that's clearly what it was, I began screengrabbing the tweets, wondering if they would be taken down later. It turns out, I was right.

There were a significant number of Twitter accounts discussing the night in question, and others posturing that if their friends got in trouble for this they were going to be "pissed." Girls were calling the victim a whore, and I was absolutely overwhelmed at the amount of information that was put out on the Internet by the time I went to bed that afternoon.

I literally was up all night saving screenshots and taking notes. With each student account I read, the more horrified I was. It was very difficult for me to even comprehend that anyone could be this callous—let alone a child.

After the first blog post I did, I got a surge of traffic on the Steubenville story. People in town were seeking out information about the case because the media was not providing the information about the critical role social media had played in the case.

During my research, I had also discovered evidence of a second assault that took place last April. Nodianos actually makes reference to the "rape at Palooza" in his twelve-minute video. I started posting screenshots on my blog from the various Twitter accounts, and that is when people really became enraged.

It is one thing to hear the rumors, but I think when people actually saw the tweets, and the vile things that were said, with their own eyes, it really drove home just how disgusting the behavior of these kids was that night.

Soon locals began contacting me stating that they believed there was a cover-up into investigation of the charges. That's not a new allegation for Steubenville. There is also a belief among residents of Steubenville that high school athletes are given a pass when it comes to accountability for bad behavior.

My articles were based on my firsthand knowledge of the area, as well as many, many emails from residents seeking to dissect truth from gossip. EVERYONE in town was talking about this case. My blog became the Internet version of a local coffee shop where people could anonymously discuss theories and other information they had heard, but their ultimate yearning was that the truth be revealed. They were concerned that the students would be given leniency because of who they were and how they were connected to the football program.

There were rumors that Coach Reno Saccoccia knew about the incident and rather than benching the students involved he allowed them to continue their football season minus one game—and later during trial testimony we were to find out that this was true.

Having lived in Steubenville, I have personal knowledge of the football culture there. I saw it—I experienced it and to be honest, I was creeped out by it. Men who were twenty years out of high school seemed to be still living in the moment of when the full-capacity stadium used to cheer loudly for them. Perhaps they are holding on to the days when they were admired and adulated, only to grow up and be stuck in a town that now has few jobs and little to do other than head back to that elaborate 10,000-seat stadium on Friday nights and relive their glory days.

If you ask any little boy in Steubenville what he wants to be when he grows up, you will likely hear "a Big Red football player." Student athletes have referred to themselves on Twitter as "#steubenvillestarsforlife."

They didn't just decide one day that they were superstars. This is a culture that has bred this attitude, and it is not well received when people discuss it critically. A quick read of some of the local high school football forums will introduce you to the rivalry between the various local high school teams. So, when I talked about the football culture negatively in light of this case, to say it was not received well is an understatement.

I never expected this case to take on the life that it has. I have been left weeping and filled with so much pride as I watched the Steubenville rallies and listened to the stories of other victims who were too afraid to come forward. It was absolutely amazing to see the streets of downtown Steubenville filled with supporters from all over the country supporting Jane Doe—and all Jane Does.

I have received emails from around the world by people who have been moved by this case in some form or another. This case has created a social awareness about rape culture, and it has opened dialogues between parents and their children that it's okay to be the lone man standing as long as you STAND.

It has forced parents to become more informed about how their children are using social media and how detrimental ones' digital footprint can be, and it has given people an opportunity to speak out against injustice.

It has been a long, tumultuous and oftentimes agonizing journey that came with great cost to my family and myself personally and physically. My family and I are no different than others. We have feelings and compassion, unlike so many who stood by and chose to do nothing that night—or the adults who revictimized Jane Doe by making excuses for the abhorrent behavior of their own children.

I was targeted for speaking of that which should not be spoken, and as I sit here writing this, Jane Doe is receiving not only death threats from locals, but is also being maligned by Big Red students because their friends were convicted.

THIS is the sort of behavior that has caused the world outside of the Big Red bubble to recoil in disgust.

And it's what has caused my world to be turned upside down.

I continued to cover the case on my blog, which had turned into a town hall of sorts. In October, I received a phone call from a friend and my "hello" was answered with, "Did you get sued?" I had no clue what my friend was talking about and I laughed and I said no. Jokingly I asked, "What did I do now?"

She told me that WTOV9 had just announced on the news that myself and twenty-five anonymous commenters from my blog were being sued for defamation of character. I think I laughed because I was shocked that anyone would file a defamation suit—especially since the lawsuit was filed by the man who it turns out was Jane Doe's ex-boyfriend and tweeted the now infamous photo of her appearing lifeless and being carried like an animal.

My friends took to social media to tweet about the defamation case, and through the amazing Ken White and popehat.com I was able to assemble an amazing team of lawyers to assist in my defense of the right to free speech: Thomas Haren, Jeffrey Nye, and Marc Randazza. I was so worried about my anonymous commenters being retaliated against if their identities were revealed.

I spent countless hours emailing or on the phone reassuring them that we were going to get through this. I wasn't going to leave them hanging, but I wasn't going to go down without a fight either. We all had the right to talk about this case—and I wanted to protect that right. Through the awesomeness of my attorneys, we were able to involve the Ohio chapter of the ACLU to represent all of the John Doe defendants and the lawsuit was dismissed with prejudice on December 27, 2012.

Hatred is a very negative waste of time, however, it hasn't stopped a small group of citizens of Steubenville from unleashing their fury upon me—all for standing up for the defenseless Jane Doe on that horrible night that changed her life forever.

I have been called a "slut," a "drunk," a "bitch with an agenda," a "liar" and someone who hates Big Red so bad that my desire was to bring down their football program. I was accused in a letter to the editor in the local paper as using my blog as a vehicle which "has lent itself to character assassination and has begun to resemble a lynch mob."

I was hospitalized for a week in November by the stress of the lawsuit that exacerbated a twenty-year-old health condition, and accused of lying about it to get attention. My mother was followed around for a week by private investigators hired by the family suing me and my photo was taken to business locations in the area asking, "Have you seen her?"

My mother and brother have been harassed online, and my recently deceased stepfather's address and phone number were posted online. What is more despicable about posting his information is that he had just been in a horrible car accident, which ultimately took his life a month later.

Perhaps most ridiculously, I was accused of "complicating" the case because I posted the screen captures of content that these kids willingly posted themselves.

My best friend disavowed our friendship over this case. Imagine my utter devastation and hurt when I realized she was participating in some of the mudslinging against me. Her mother even joined the fray and used Twitter to state what a "fat sweat hog" and "bitch" I was, and how she wished I would "get AIDS and die a slow death."

So would I do it all over again? ABSOLUTELY.

The verdict is finally in, but this story is far from over. The Ohio Attorney General's office has ordered a grand jury to convene in April 2013 to investigate additional charges against others.

Today is one that is filled with many emotions: joy that Jane Doe is able to move on with her life now; sadness and compassion for all of the lives that were forever changed because of a night of bad decisions, and contempt for those who did nothing to stop this terrible chain of events. Because at the end of the day, the only agenda I have is simple.

Let's prevent another Jane Doe from happening ever again. Let's comfort the ones brave enough to stand up in the face of adversity. And let's encourage all the Jane Does too afraid to come forward to have renewed strength and courage in the wake of the Steubenville verdict.

Because you are not alone.

Porn Director: I Changed My Mind about Condoms

Nica Noelle

"My chlamydia and gonorrhea test results aren't back yet," a nineteen-year-old I'll call Cheryl said in a raspy whisper, her small hand covering her cell phone as the nurse at the clinic waited on the other end.

"Well, when do they think the results will be in?" I asked, trying not to sound panicked. My entire cast and crew was in the next room waiting for the results, which would clear her to perform hardcore sex on camera with a male costar.

"Probably not until Monday," Cheryl said. "I'm so sorry, Nica."

"Fuck," I whispered, walking into one of the dark, empty rooms on the soundstage. "Fuck, fuck, fuck."

I was already several thousand dollars over budget due to production disasters and "no call/no show" performers. It was crucial that I finish the movie, but by law, there was only one way I could allow Cheryl to perform a sex scene without a current STD test: by allowing her costar to wear a condom.

I'd been told many times that condoms in porn meant certain death to sales. Conventional wisdom suggested that nobody wants condoms in their sexual fantasy. Porn was supposed to be an escape, not a public service announcement or a reminder that sex is dangerous or risky.

This was prior to 2012, when the controversial Measure B made condoms mandatory in porn—a law recently upheld, though it is still being fought by adult film producers who believe it's catastrophic to our industry. For a long time I agreed with them, and though I've long struggled with the subject, here's how much I didn't want a condom in my film that day: I replaced Cheryl.

Actually, it was the president of the parent company who made that decision, but I'm the one who accepted it and had to break the news to Cheryl, who was surprisingly gracious about it. I'd come to porn hoping to change the way it was made, but that day, I felt like a scumbag.

I compare my career ascension in porn to falling into the rabbit hole, à la *Alice in Wonderland*. While working as a litigation paralegal and moonlighting as a journalist seven years ago, I got an assignment to write about the making of a fetish video. In order to do the job right, I decided to audition for a role in a spanking video and perform in it myself.

The experience was life changing: instead of feeling degraded, I'd left the shoot feeling oddly euphoric and—even more oddly— empowered. I began working for other adult film studios, including a small, unknown lesbian porn company whose owner operated out of his modest Encino, California, home. After using me as a model for several shoots, he offered me a job as creative director. My mission, he explained, was to transform his company from a niche studio into the "leader in lesbian erotica." It meant quitting my job at the law firm and taking a huge pay cut, but I felt destiny knocking. Within a year, the studio was the talk of the adult industry and I was being hailed as a trailblazer in a "new era" of adult films.

And so, along with "suburban mom," "journalist" and "paralegal," I added "pornographer" (a label I proudly, defiantly claimed) to my résumé. My overnight success gave me the confidence (or was it arrogance?) to think I might change not only what kind of movies fans watched but also how adult performers would be treated on set.

I'd heard stories of performers forced to have sex on dirt roads and in back alleys, on dirty carpets infested with fleas, and on semen-stained couches. I'd heard tales of porn "stars" being denied access to soap and showers, and given no food or drinks after twelve or more hours on set. Most adult performers also accepted as par for the course that they'd be sexually harassed not only by producers but also the lowliest members of the studio's production crew.

Not on my set. It was time to borrow a playbook from the corporate environment I'd left behind.

My first rule: No one on my crew can "hit on" the talent. I explained to them that doing so places the performer in a tricky position, much like when a boss asks his secretary out and she agrees for fear of losing her job.

"Our performers are naked, and you are clothed," I reminded my bewildered crew. "You're in a position of authority, and you're not to abuse it." This rule made me instantly unpopular with male crew members, but I didn't care. If they broke it more than once, they were fired.

Another rule: Nude performers would never be told to sit, lie down or perform sex acts on unwashed or unprotected surfaces. Counters and desktops would be thoroughly washed with antibacterial soap or spray, and beds and couches would have clean linens—either straight from the washing machine or brand-new from the store (I provided these myself). It was alarming how strange and even unreasonable my crew found these requests to be, despite the fact that staph infection was a constant problem on adult film sets and performers routinely canceled shoots citing a "spider bite." ("Spider bite" had become something of a euphemism for "staph infection" in the adult industry.)

But the one thing I didn't insist on was condoms. It was a given that we didn't use them; that's what our mandatory thirty-day STD tests were for. It was the "industry standard," and while I didn't hesitate to question other industry standards that might place performers in harm's way (or just create an unpleasant environment), for some reason the condom issue sounded no alarms for me.

Perhaps that's partially because I'm allergic to latex myself. If I have sex with a man who's wearing a latex condom, within twenty-four hours of the encounter I'll be in the throes of a painful urinary tract infection requiring powerful antibiotics. In my off-camera sex life I rely on STD tests, so why not rely on them at work, too? I'd performed in adult films myself and felt fine about simply verifying my scene partner's current, negative STD test.

But there may have been a deeper, darker reason for my refusal to consider the question of condoms. While I've always said I wasn't in porn for the money, the truth was that as my success grew I was increasingly concerned with career failure. I wanted my movies to keep selling, and on a practical level, I wanted to continue paying my rent and my child's school tuition. I had worked hard to get where I was, damn it, and I wanted to build on that success, not sabotage it.

Which is of course what happens to many people who finally "make it." They start drifting from the values and ideals they once stood for, and which may have even directly resulted in their success. I cherished the image I'd built of caring about performers' welfare, but if "taking it too far" was going to threaten my chance to stay in business, why not just hide behind the old way of doing things? Why was I so hell-bent on being a saint? I suddenly (conveniently) wondered.

I actually kept a box of condoms on set in case a performer should request one. I'd assembled "hygiene kits" filled with items like baby wipes, shampoo, tampons, nail clippers, deodorant, douches and spermicide, so why not include condoms, just in case? But on the rare occasions a performer asked for one, I felt anxiety, even as I smiled and handed one over: Would I get in trouble with my studio for allowing it? What would it mean for sales? Why was the performer asking for a condom, anyway—didn't she know it was a "condom-free" shoot? Why didn't she tell me she had issues with it before accepting the role?

So, when the Measure B "condom law" was passed in November 2012, I loudly objected, along with thousands of other adult industry producers. Measure B was both dangerous and absurd, we argued. First of all, our testing system works, we reasoned, because we had successfully kept HIV out of the talent pool since 2004. Secondly, the condom law would simply force pornographers "underground," where they could no longer be monitored or held accountable for violations in safety protocol (as if everyone in porn was already held accountable for any number of random, unethical behaviors). Our hard-won testing standards would erode as performers opted not to share their STD test results, or even to test at all. And not only that, what if the condom were to break and you didn't know your scene partner's HIV status? What if you were (like me) allergic to condoms and the condom law would end your career as a performer?

I made these arguments more than once, and I believed them, but on a deeper, quieter level, I felt conflicted. What I knew was that, despite the validity of these "what if?" scenarios, and despite the fact that our testing system had been successful at keeping HIV out of the porn talent pool for nearly a decade, it had been far less successful in keeping out other STDs. I knew that condoms would help prevent the spread of diseases like chlamydia and gonorrhea, both of which are so common in the adult industry that a performer who learns he or she is infected doesn't even bother to alert recent scene partners to their possible exposure. And while porn's most commonly transmitted STDs are admittedly "curable" with a course of antibiotics, they can still have some fairly serious complications (e.g., infertility and increased vulnerability to the HIV virus).

I also couldn't help noticing that while some performers seemed all but immune to porn's most common STDs, others seemed to struggle with "dirty tests" constantly. I knew this because sometimes I'd try to book a certain performer only to be told by her agent that she wasn't available until she could "take her medicine and retest." Even if I'd been told the same thing about the same performer multiple times within the span of a few months, I wouldn't miss a beat. "Tell me when she's up and running again," I'd say, and simply ask if one of my alternate choices was available instead. While I was vigilant about keeping my set staph-and-sexual-harassment-free, apparently chronic cases of chlamydia and gonorrhea—some of which might have very well been transmitted on my set—didn't faze me.

But after a few heavily publicized HIV scares in the past few years, including four within the past few weeks (none of which turned out to have been contracted on set, nor transmitted to other adult film performers in the course of shooting a scene), it has become harder for many of us to avoid the question of whether condoms might not be such a bad idea. In terms of sales they're risky, but when considering performer safety, is there really a solid argument against a testing/condom combination? Yes, some producers might continue to shoot condom-free porn anyway, but is that any excuse for the rest of us to avoid taking steps to protect our performers?

Now, as the president of my own production company (which partners with the online broadcasting network AEBN.net), I've been given an opportunity to follow my own conscience and to control my own career and financial future. Should I refuse to bow to "the Man" and go underground like many of my peers have already started to do? Shoot without legal film permits and operate in the shadows? Or do I search my soul for truths that don't stem from a need to rebel against authority or protect my own bottom line?

I've concluded I want my performers to be safe more than I want to be "the most successful porn director." I want them to leave my set feeling good about participating in my movie and to never look back on it with regret. I don't want them to experience a surge of fear and shame when they learn their next STD test results. And most of all I don't want to encourage them to be nonchalant about their health.

"What if?" arguments aside, condoms, along with a current,

valid STD test, will do a pretty good job of ensuring that performers on my set will go home without anything new to worry about. Are condoms foolproof? No. Neither is an STD test, even if it's a very recent one. But would requiring condoms and a test make for a safer work environment? Yes—by a very wide margin.

But what if nobody buys my "condom porn" movies? What if my competitors continue to shoot "bareback sex" in secret locations, avoiding detection and forcing me out of business?

That's a possibility I fear. But nowhere near as much as I fear exposing already vulnerable, stigmatized performers to preventable STDs on my set. Not as much as I fear being directly responsible for a performer's inability to pay their rent as I go on paying mine, indifferent to their struggle. I don't want to live that life. I don't want to be that person.

Yet, I do believe there are valid First Amendment arguments in favor of condom-free porn. As an artist it bothers me that I can no longer film completely nude bodies or "all natural," explicit lovemaking, even when shooting monogamous, married couples. It bothers me that those of us with allergies to condoms will not be accommodated and will be completely shut out of performing. I believe there should be room for accommodations; there should be exceptions made if, for example, adherence to certain rigid health and safety standards can be verified. Just as mainstream directors are allowed to put actors and stunt people at increased risk as long as increased safety protocols are followed, a similar provision could apply to the adult industry so that we might maintain our right to freedom of artistic expression. (Some of us do actually venture to make art, believe it or not.)

But the catch is, we have to prove we're responsible enough to follow such rigid safety standards and to take rules and laws seriously. (Not just those we "want" to follow or have imposed on ourselves.) We have to show we can operate within the law and not angrily threaten to break it when there's a ruling we don't like. We have to demonstrate that we care about the health of those we work with more than we care about making a quick, sleazy buck. If we want legal rights and protections we have to accept the reality that, like any legitimate business, we will be supervised, held accountable and penalized if we don't conduct ourselves professionally—and ethically.

We have to do something that an industry obsessed with being forever young, wild and free is loath to do:

We have to grow up.

Pregger Libido
Ember Swift

When our bodies start making another human body, the process is so complex that it's no wonder we're exhausted. As this is my second pregnancy, I'm surprised that I'd forgotten this fact. I'm currently six months along and so for the past half a year, I've found myself wanting to nod off at 10:00 p.m. or falling asleep the moment my head hits the pillow. Although, this time, I also have a toddler who still wakes me up at night to go "pee pee," but sleep mercifully returns quickly after that task is done. Sleep has become my most steady companion.

When I was pregnant with my first child—my daughter—I was equally exhausted, but this also permeated my mood, which in turn permeated my libido. I don't think pregnant women speak often enough with each other about how pregnancy hormones affect libido.

I was shy to admit to my friends (especially those who had

had children or who were also pregnant) that I was absolutely not interested in having any kind of marital relations with my husband. There were occasional exceptions to that state of mind, but it's truthful to say that our intimacy levels dropped substantially during my first pregnancy. This embarrassed me. I feared others would think I was punishing our partnership for what was happening to my body. I was also afraid that I had forgotten how to connect with the person I loved. Thankfully, after the birth of our daughter, things went back to a relative normal.

With baby number one, I also did all my previous prenatal care in China and we were advised early on to avoid sexual relations for health and safety reasons. Chinese doctors are notoriously discreet in this regard and so the rationale was vague at best. In the West, the necessity for abstinence during pregnancy—even during the first trimester—has long been disproved. In fact, having intimate relations with our partners is now encouraged by Western doctors. Both the rocking motion and the hormones generated through pleasure are comforting to the growing fetus.

Regardless of knowing this more modern information from the West, during my daughter's gestation I was quite happy to adhere to the old-fashioned practices advocated in China. In a conservative country, I opportunistically became conservative myself—an excellent veil for what more accurately was just an absentee libido.

Now, fast-forward to baby number two. I am a fine example of the saying, "every pregnancy is different." I am not as emotionally exhausted, I'm in a brighter and better mood, and I have a strangely *elevated* sex drive. More desire, less darkness. I am receiving my prenatal care in Canada and now it is my partner's turn to opportunistically adhere to more liberal Western practices. In other words, it's time for him to accommodate the demands of my growing libido!

This is where you are anticipating a happy ending. You might expect to read that my husband and I have been having wonderful, wild sex throughout this second child's gestation. This piece will have successfully solicited both congratulatory nods and hints of reader envy. Maybe I should quit while I'm ahead....

Alas, truth is my model and so I must confess that ever since my belly has become visible, he's hesitated, unsure as to whether he wants to have "sex with his son."

What?! I have been hard on him about this, arguing that my body is still my body, my "needs" are still my "needs," and his son is never going to remember his father in any compromising position. He still hesitates (but usually complies). Sometimes I truly feel like the stereotypical man in this partnership; it's the first time I've had to convince him to go to bed with me. Geesh.

This mysterious situation never had the opportunity to present itself during my first pregnancy because I simply wasn't interested. How many other pregnant women have found themselves feeling horny only to be confronted with their "freaked out" partner who is concerned about the connection between the child and sex? Or their fear of hurting the baby or crushing the baby in the act, et cetera? Where is the line between being a woman and being a mother? Does our sex appeal disappear as soon as our bellies swell? These are questions I may never know the answers to. As I mentioned, we pregger ladies aren't talking about this enough.

As a saving grace, my husband's hesitation has found a peaceful perch between my elevated exhaustion and elevated libido. When sleep has become my greatest companion, do I even have the energy to convince my partner that he's missing out? And for myself, when I can't keep my eyes open in bed, how are my desires going to get fulfilled? I've proposed several creative solutions, not to fear, and he's intrigued by my persistence. I'm too shy to write about them here, however. Wish us luck.

But, as a final commentary, I believe strongly that as our pregnant female bodies change, get larger, get unrecognizable—especially the first time it happens—it's so important to push ourselves to allow our partners to love us, to touch us, to celebrate our body's new shape and growth. Often, our addition of a baby bump makes us even more beautiful and sexy to those who love us, even when we don't believe it.

If, like me in my first pregnancy, our libidos have left through the same door as our entire wardrobe, we women nonetheless have to push ourselves to stay open to letting our bodies be loved. There are lots of options in this regard. Massage, being bathed, or allowing our partners to rub oils or skin cream into the rising globe of our baby bellies enables our loved ones to stay connected to our physical changes, not to mention gives us another (non-sexual) outlet to staying physically connected with them.

This time, I'm doing better at remembering these things and celebrating my body.

But first, I must sleep. At this very second in time, sleep is the *sexiest* bedmate!

The White Kind of Body
Alok Vaid-Menon

A couple of years ago I performed a poem about my internalized racism and how it shapes my sexual desires. After the performance several people approached me in private and confessed that they, too, had grown up with white fetish, but never felt comfortable articulating that publicly. Since then I have traveled across the world sharing my poetry and facilitating workshops about desire, capitalism, and colonialism. Everywhere I go there is always that similar moment of confession: *I feel the same way.*

Race, it seems, structures our desires just as much—if not more—than gender. As queer people of color we find ourselves struggling to make sense of our identities and desires with the language of sexual identity politics that was never meant for us. In this piece I want to share my personal story as a queer South Asian growing up and show how the ways we have come to talk about sexuality perpetuate white supremacy. It is my hope that by (re)turning to our personal narratives—rather than merely adopting prescribed sexual identities—we can begin to imagine new ways of talking about sexuality, power, and identity that center racial justice.

Coming Out (White)

The mainstream gay narrative often requires a story that begins with trauma, abjection, and insecurity and ends with liberation, visibility, and confidence. We are asked: When did you know? When did you first figure it out? And we respond with the stories they want to hear: we tell them about screaming "I'm gay" outside in the middle of the night, we tell them about sneaking looks in the locker room, about that perpetual fear of being found out. But we do not tell them about the first time we were called a terrorist. We do not tell them about how we refused to speak our native tongue at home. These gay coming out stories privilege the trauma that comes from being a sexual minority, but they rarely hold space for the inherent violence of navigating the world with a body that is not white. For a culture so invested in notions of authenticity and visibility, the silence around racial justice from white queer people is revealing.

The truth is I have always been attracted to whiteness. I remember in kindergarten I would develop crushes on all the white boys in my class—those white boys who came from rich families with mothers who ran the parent-teacher organizations, those white boys who played Little League baseball and joined Boy Scouts. I'm talking about *that* kind of whiteness: that accumulation of culture and class that every immigrant is fed as representative of the American Dream.

These were the days I would go home and ask my mother why we didn't go to church. I would tell my grandmother to stop wearing *saris* and put on pants instead. These were the days I'd ask my parents *why we weren't like other families*: why we didn't eat steak for dinner, and watch football, and do the things that *normal families do*. Growing up I always felt inadequate and embarrassed by my Brownness and my Hindu culture. I would willingly attend Christian youth groups with my white friends and feel so much more validation from their acceptance than from the elders in my own community.

This attraction was always about power. I wanted to be white so desperately because that meant I would finally be normal, finally be accepted. I admired the white boys in my kindergarten class because they had power, they had respect, they were *beautiful*.

When you are a Brown kid in the South you are never given the language to articulate your constant feelings of inadequacy. There is no lesson, there are no textbooks, there is no acknowledgment of your struggle. There is just the unbearable whiteness of being that swallows you whole and you hope that you are spit out still alive. It was only after 9/11 that I gained access to a word that finally described the distance between me and my classmates: race.

I remember it vividly: on September 12 my mother told me to be careful at school. My middle school had an assembly in the gym. We were all instructed to wear red, white, and blue and we gathered and sang the national anthem. I remember singing as loud as the rest, and I remember feeling part of something bigger than myself. I didn't really understand what happened, but goddamnit I knew that I was American. I knew it in the same way my Hindu temple knew that it was a good idea to put an American flag on the back of our T-shirts: God bless America / we will never forget September 11. After the assembly a white classmate came up to me and asked me, "Why did *your* people do this to *us?*" And for the first time everything made sense. The lines were drawn in the sand. I was Brown and they were white and there was nothing I could do about it.

The truth is, at some level, I began to believe everything they said. I began to believe that I was not an American. I began to believe that my people were guilty. And in the deepest parts of myself I began to believe that my people were ugly for it.

Coming into consciousness of my Brownness occurred at the same time I began to come into awareness of my queerness. It's impossible for me to divorce these narratives—they have been, and will always be—interrelated. The boys I began to fantasize about were the same boys I wrote love letters to as a child, were the same boys I wanted so desperately to become. The boys—the men—I was sexually attracted to were the very white men who made me feel ugly, made me feel insignificant, made me feel worthless.

In some ways, my queerness *worked as a mechanism of my racial oppression and contributed to my feelings of racial inadequacy*. Now, the very white men who degraded me felt *sexy* to me. My desire shackled me to white supremacy. As much as I wanted to love my Brownness—I became *even more* drawn to, tantalized by, and attracted to whiteness. As much as I resented the racial trauma inflicted by the white men around me, I found myself deeply attracted to them. I found myself accepting their insults, their stereotypes, their constant racism—excusing it because at least they were paying attention to me. This is how insidious white supremacy is: it will not only terrorize you, but will make you desire your own oppression. How are you supposed to escape from a nightmare when it feels like a wet dream?

When I "came out" and began to consume queer media—pornography, blogs, movies, et cetera—the depictions of queerness upheld white supremacy. Queer characters were almost always white, gay porn almost always included white cisgender men—

unless it was explicitly marked as interracial or racial fetish. At first I didn't mind this. In fact, I enjoyed it; I found these depictions of whiteness seductive.

The representation of queer life on the screen proved to be fairly accurate when I moved to the Bay Area in California and finally had access to other queer people. Almost everyone was white. Nonetheless, I threw myself in headfirst, joining every political group and attending every function I possibly could. Now that I look back on it, consuming this media, coming out as "gay," and organizing within a traditional "gay rights" framework made me happy at some level because *I felt like I was becoming more white*. Being "gay," being part of a "gay" community, gave me an opportunity to escape from my race, gave me new connections to whiteness, new ways to intimately embrace it and experience its validation.

As I began to get more involved with mainstream gay life, I found myself feeling less Brown. I used language and identity-frameworks that were inaccessible to the South Asian community I grew up with. When my family didn't understand the word *queer*, rather than trying to understand where they were coming from I dismissed them as homophobic and transphobic. My white peers assured me that people of color "tended to be more traditional" and I believed them because I had to in order to sustain my delusion and our relationships. I went to parties and conferences with mostly white people who would identify me as the "minority in the room." The more time I spent in white queer communities, the more I stopped thinking about race. This didn't mean thinking about race only in the abstract, it meant that I stopped thinking about my family. I stopped thinking about my people. I became so focused on liberation for (white) queer people that I couldn't see how that didn't actually mean liberation for anyone else. White queers found any conversation about my experiences of racism going on to be an "unrelated issue," so I even fabricated a more conventional coming out story to fit in. This is how effortlessly white supremacy works: it appropriates and distorts our own narratives and bodies into its own image before we even recognize how this might be affecting the rest of our people.

There Is No Brown in Your Rainbow

In queer communities I began to hear people talk about how validating their relationships with other queers were. There seemed to be this idea that all heterosexual relationships were inherently oppressive no matter what and that, in contrast, queer relationships were subversive.

The truth is my first and most transformative relationship was with a woman my first year of high school. She was South Asian. We started getting close after we shared our experiences with racial trauma, our experiences as diasporic Indians, and our anxieties about our Hindu religion in our small town. Our subsequent relationship was perhaps one of the most significant journeys for my path toward self-actualization. I began to feel beauty in Brownness, to not be ashamed of who I was and where I came from. Looking back, I was less attracted to her gender, *and more attracted to her race.* Dominant ideas of heterosexuality suggest that cis men enter relationships with the "opposite" gender. Heterosexuality is understood as an attraction to *difference.* But this model could not hold my intense desire for this woman. I was attracted to her because of our mutual sameness, not our difference. But at the time I did not have the language to explain what was going on. I grew up thinking that if you had desire for men like I did you had to be gay. So I told her that we could never be together.

My first queer relationships didn't seem to live up to all they were built up to be. In all of my subsequent relationships with white men, I was unable to experience a sense of solidarity and kinship. Dominant narratives of homosexuality describe it as "same-sex" desire: we hear stories about how men *"know how to please other men better because they have a penis."* We hear how same-sex relationships are more functional because both parties "get one another." These ideas never really seemed to make sense to me. All of my relationships with white men have felt much more conflicted, racially charged, and oppositional. Embracing a white male body never feels comfortable, natural, *same*. It feels foreign.

As I began to participate in (white) queer communities I recognized that what attracted to me to these boys—what had always attracted me to whiteness—was its difference from me. Whiteness was a commodity, a property that I didn't own and was systematically denied. I wanted to be with white guys because I was attracted to their power. I found myself turning down incredibly charming queer people of color, because I just didn't get the same power trip.

My early and uncritical experiences with white men reminded me that I can never have access to this cultural capital, that I will always be Brown, no matter how much queers profess to be "one community." I began to realize the extreme racism and colorism that governs much of queer life (especially for queer men): the lighter you are, the more attractive you are. The darker you are, the more likely you are to be friend-zoned.

The majority of the times I found myself invisible to the white queer gaze. I met white boys with dating profiles that read: *No Asians/No Fems*. Sexual racism and femmephobia like this was rarely as explicit; it manifested itself in more silent and pernicious ways: always being the "friend" and never anything more. When I would confront my white queer friends about why they didn't date people of color they'd often say things like: "I don't see race—get over it, it's not important!" And though they would often profess liberal and antiracist politics, they would still only sleep with and date other white cis men. When I began to meet white queer men who did date across the color line they would often say that race wasn't central to their desire or relationship. The idea was that being gay already involved transgressing one taboo, why not jump over another? I heard this narrative a lot: queer desire is inherently transgressive so therefore it is somehow exempt from complicity.

Those white queer men who did express interest in people of color often articulated it in ways that were just as problematic, just in a reverse direction. One white boy told me that he had always wanted to be with a Brown man. He told me that I felt like a *real* man (disregarding how I identified). And, at the time, I not only accepted it, I fetishized it. For the first time in my life I experienced validation from the very body that taunted me growing up. I performed my race—in its most stereotypical forms—for him so that I could maintain his desire. In subsequent relationships I experienced similar fetishization. It manifested itself in sometimes subtle ways—comments on my rugged masculinity (gesturing to histories of associations with bodies of color and primitive animality) and cloaked racist sayings like "all South Asians are so sexy" (as if one sixth of the world's population looks the same).

In all of these experiences—the ones where I was hyper invisible and hyper visible—one theme remained constant: I was always reduced to my race. My race was the primary basis of my desirability or undesirability. I never was able to enter interactions where my race was not salient—the paradigm established was that I was always the one with "the race," while whiteness remained unmarked.

After severally racially charged experiences with white men

I found myself in some of the deepest and most visceral racial trauma of my life. I found myself predicating my very self-worth on validation from white men. It didn't matter how many people of color were attracted to me, only white guys counted. It didn't matter to me how successful I was in school or how effective of an activist I was, only validation by white men could make me happy. What had begun as a survival strategy—fetishizing the very white men who made my life miserable in high school as a way to establish a sense of control at least in the realm of fantasy—ended up becoming a nightmare. This is how white supremacy operates: it offers you a promise of acceptance, always at a distance, so that you are always running after it. It is always an abusive dynamic: it creates dynamics where your entire self worth is predicated on the very people who hurt you the most.

There came a point in my life when I could not longer submit myself to the constant humiliation of arguing for my humanity to the very men who oppressed me. It might sound dramatic but there is something deeply personal about sexual intimacy—especially for those of us who have grown up our entire lives being told that we are ugly. It was never about a date or a hookup, it was always about my worth is as a human being. I realized that I needed a more sustainable way to develop self-worth. Like so many people of color before me I sought refuge in my own. I began to build intentional community with other queer people of color and it was in these spaces that I experienced the healing justice I had always longed for. I recognized how my attraction to whiteness was linked to my own racial self-hatred. I recognized the ways in which desire for whiteness helps justify the continued subordination of my peoples. I finally felt part of spaces that held me in my entirety. Slowly I have begun to unhinge my sexuality from whiteness and expand the horizon of my desires. Naturally it's a process, but I have finally begun to feel like I have control of my desires and I'd like to think that means something in a world determined to relinquish control from people of color.

Somewhere Over the Rainbow

My story is similar to those of so many queer and trans people of color. We each have our own unique experiences of being disenfranchised by queer communities, but across the board we express our collective grief and rage at how queerness has come to signify whiteness. So many of us have never been able to disassociate our racial oppression from our gender and sexual oppression. The idea of seeing these as separate struggles not only feels inconsiderate, it feels deliberately misleading and violent. Yet, race neutrality and outright racial hostility continues to persist in queer white spaces and progressive sexuality spaces more generally. Many queers continue to organize, fuck, make art, dream, and build together in ways that do not actively address white supremacy. It is important to establish that this is not about ignorance; this is about power.

Race neutrality is not a passive act; it is a conscious act of prejudice. The refusal to engage with race is actually an acceptance of white supremacy. In our "postracial" and neoliberal moment racism actually operates by white people and other privileged people proclaiming that "race has nothing to do with." What I have tried to demonstrate with my story is that the supposed universality of sexual identity politics actually masks over racism. Sexual identity politics only map well onto the experiences of white privileged people because they were made for them. I am not advocating for the inclusion of race into sexual identity politics. To do so would be to imply that racism is the exception, and not the norm. Rather, I am suggesting that we need fundamentally different ways of talking about and organizing around desire. I'd like to close with several suggestions that we can consider moving forward.

1. We need to stop expecting conversations about race and sexuality to only be had by people of color. To do so is to suggest that race only belongs to people of color and therefore to leave whiteness unchecked.
Race should not just be the intellectual and political preoccupation of people of color. White people also have a race. Whiteness has the privilege to be unmarked, especially when it comes to sexuality politics. While it might not be as immediately explicit, white people have also had their desires and identities mediated by their race. White people who are in relationships with other white people are still actively creating and engaging in race. Indeed, white fetish is not just a peculiar phenomenon found among people of color, rather it is the dominant framing of a world where whiteness is marketed as desirable. It should not be controversial or stigmatized to talk about racial fetish; it should be a practice we all engage in. None of us are somehow outside of white supremacy. White supremacy is a system and we experience its symptoms every single day. Our assumption should be that any idea or politics expressed in a racist society is going to be shaped by racist values. It is only until we can *name* racism that we can begin to have conversations about how to confront it. If you expect people of color to always be the ones to bring up race then actually you are making people of color do all the labor (and where have we seen that before!).

2. There is nothing inherently progressive about queer sexual identity or relationships. Relying on an equation

that positions queer relationships as somehow more "subversive" than "heterosexual" relationships is racist. Queer people often present themselves as more progressive than the average "straight" person because they are "less conservative." Yet this binary between "conservative" and "progressive" masks over how both of these groups are complicit in white supremacy. Oppression is not just a feeling or attitude; it is a system of power. False dichotomies between "progressive" and "conservative" distract us from having real conversations about structural complicity. There is nothing really progressive about a politics of sexuality alone. Sexual identity politics has done the remarkable act of creating norms in which we are not allowed to question people's desires or relationships because they are somehow "personal." The political act in sexual identity politics is announcing or declaring one's sexuality. Once this is accomplished one is magically outside of any scrutiny. This leaves us no space to comment on the oppressive forces at work when white cis men only sleep with other white cis men. Only focusing on gender without attention to race results in always positioning white people as more progressive. The real work of any politics around sexuality shouldn't be just the articulation of our desires, but also the tough conversations about power and desire and the even more difficult task of transforming our desires.

3. Anchoring sexual identity to gender/sex object choice alone is racist.

The dominant understanding of sexual identity is that our identities are linked to the "sex" we are attracted to. Along with the inherent transphobia in such a paradigm, it is important to establish that the only people in this world who have the privilege to understand their sex/gender outside of race are white people.

Therefore, to establish that sexual orientation is solely about "gender" or "sex" (as if these things exist outside of race) is to perpetuate white supremacy. "Men" and "women" do not exist as stable and oppositional categories when you take into account racial and gender identity, and other various registers of difference. When we experience attraction it is not only due to sex or gender, it is also due to a host of other factors (class, race, education status, et cetera.) If we only narrate our identities through gender object choice we aren't actually being honest about how power operates. The privileging of sex/gender in the ways that we discuss desire is not just coincidental, it is a carefully crafted strategy to maintain racial dominance.

4. We should no longer speak about desire and preference as if they exist outside of systems of power.

People are not born beautiful; they become beautiful because they have access to power. We live in a world that constantly teaches us that the very people who control the world (white cis able-bodied men) are the most attractive people. We are taught to fetishize whiteness and masculinity because our desire helps fuel our own subordination. Therefore the idea that our desires are somehow fixed or innate and cannot be changed over time is also about saying that racial and gender inequality in this world can never be changed. We must stop pretending that our sexual and romantic preferences are somehow separate from the material distribution of power in this world. We must stop pretending that sexual and romantic desire somehow exists outside of the other desires for power, wealth, property, and conquest. We must stop pretending as if we do not inherit our desires from histories of colonialism and contemporary white supremacy. We cannot ever fully disintegrate our individual wants from what we have been told to desire. We need to become more comfortable speaking about the ways in which all of our desires are implicated in these violent systems and how we actively (re)create power through exercising our desires.

5. We should stop prescribing identities and narratives for people and instead allow them to self-determine their own narratives.

What is, I think, both tremendously intimidating and exciting about sexuality is that when we take seriously how unique each one of our life histories is and how deeply our attractions and identities are linked to these histories, we recognize that no one word or identity can ever hold the complexity. Moving beyond sexual identity isn't just about postmodern intellectual radicalism, it's actually about doing what makes the most sense. Sexual identities do not actually adequately describe *anyone*; they are short signifiers that are more reductive than they are generative. What I hope we can do as people invested in sexual liberation is create more spaces for people to be more than a word or an identity. I want more spaces where people can speak honestly about all of the trauma we have experienced and discuss the ways in which our histories of violence (or lack thereof) have mediated our desires. I want us to stop attempting to categorize, label, and contain all of our pluralities. I want us to be able to embrace the chaos that comes from really doing meaningful introspective work on our desires without falling into the trap of identity. The idea of categorizing our sexuality into discrete identities is a colonial phenomenon. This process of challenging sexual identity politics and allowing a space to self-narrate our desires and identities is part of a greater struggle against white supremacy.

Sex, Lies and Public Education
Lynn Comella

What are Nevada high school students learning about sex, and how are they learning it? We talked to a few local graduates to find out.

Veronica grew up in a Catholic household where sex was never discussed except when her parents told her, "Don't have it."

In tenth grade, while attending Vo-Tech (now known as Southeast Career Technical Academy), she had a semester-long health class taught by one of the school's athletic coaches. "He was a very nice man, but he sat at his desk and put in videos," says Veronica, one of a group of young women I interviewed about their experiences with sex education.

Most of the class dealt with nutrition. When it came time for the unit on sex, the videos they watched barely covered the basics—anatomy, menstruation, hormones. Veronica's big take-away? Make sure you shower and wear deodorant.

Veronica became pregnant with her first child at eighteen, the last of her group of five high school friends to have a baby. The day she learned she was pregnant, she also learned she had a sexually transmitted infection. "I didn't know enough about birth control to use it. Eventually I learned about condoms, but nobody was using them, so I thought, 'Well, if it's okay for guys not to use them, it must be all right.'"

Today, Veronica is a thirty-two-year-old married mother of two working toward completing her undergraduate degree at UNLV. She says she can't help but wonder how her life might have been different if she had access to better information about birth control and sex.

After a bill designed to create uniform standards for sex education in Nevada public schools died in the state Senate on May 24, angry finger-pointing immediately began over who was to blame—Senate Democrats who sidestepped the issue or the bill's opponents, who argued it would advance a pro-abortion agenda.

AB230 would have required school districts to offer age-appropriate and medically accurate sex education to students, including information about safe and effective methods of contraception, gender stereotypes, negotiating healthy relationships and the prevention and treatment of sexually transmitted infections. The bill's supporters also hoped it would help reduce Nevada's teen pregnancy rate, the fourth highest in the nation.

One group, however, was conspicuously absent from much of the public discussion about the bill: students. What, I wondered, had recent Nevada high school students learned in their school-based sex education? What was discussed, what wasn't, and where did young people turn to fill in the gaps?

No Uniform Standards

While Nevada currently has statewide standards for health education, they do not include a specific set of guidelines for teaching about sex, leaving those decisions to local school districts.

"Our current regulations for sex education in Clark Country are abstinence-based, which includes medically accurate, fact-based information on contraception, pregnancy and prenatal care, fetal development and parenthood and sexually transmitted infections, including HIV and AIDS," says Shannon La Neve, K-12 health coordinator for the Clark County School District.

What students actually learn, I discovered, varies dramatically from school to school and across different school districts. And judging from the accounts of the young women I interviewed, it doesn't seem like much has changed since Veronica graduated in 1998.

"I really don't remember anything I learned from sex education in high school," Breanna, twenty-one, who graduated from Elko High School in 2009, tells me. "In middle school, they told us... well, they didn't really tell us anything except, 'Don't have sex.' In high school, it was pretty much the same thing. But you're a bunch of high school kids. You're going to want to experiment."

"I don't think we had a birth-control unit. They would show us pictures of STIs to scare us, but they never said, 'If you get an STI you have to go to a doctor; if it's herpes you have to take medication for the rest of your life but you can still have sex.' It was implied that if you got an STI your sex life was ruined."

Breanna wasn't the only person I talked to who felt that her school-based sex education was light on detailed information and heavy on scare tactics.

Maddie, seventeen, a senior at Northwest Career & Technical Academy, took a unit on drugs and date rape in eighth grade, followed by three weeks of sex education in her freshman year. She tells the same stories of a focus on STIs, complete with graphic pictures. Despite the limited information she received, she credits her health teacher for cultivating an environment where students could ask questions. But she also admits that, "Because we were so young, we weren't really sure what questions to ask."

"Honestly, I wish we would have had sex ed our junior year. Freshman year we still giggled about it. Very few kids were sexually active. I think we were still in that middle school phase. The majority of us weren't at the point in our lives to really take it in and hear about it."

"They Call It a Cookie or a Flower"

Which topics were covered in sex ed—and how they were presented—often depended on the teacher.

Maria, twenty-two, had a teacher at Cimarron Memorial High School who went beyond the district's curriculum, bringing in her own videos and other materials. She also debunked myths, like the idea that you can't get pregnant if you have sex in the shower because hot water kills sperm.

Even at the time, Maria realized her teacher was not the norm. "Her method wasn't to say, 'Don't have sex.' Rather, it was, 'If you have sex, you need to know this stuff. You need to know what is true and what is not true.' If it wasn't for her, I wouldn't have learned as much as I did."

Despite the efforts of teachers like Maria's, there are still those students who fall through the cracks. Amber, twenty-six, graduated from Bonanza High School in 2005, yet says she "somehow missed sex ed."

"I kept waiting for an opportunity to take it—it was something I was interested in—but it was never an option."

Instead, Amber eventually turned to friends and Planned Parenthood to pick up the slack. "[Clark County School District] failed me as a student. I think in Las Vegas, there's a lot of access to a lot of different things than if I lived elsewhere. I could go to an Adult Superstore to get the education I needed without getting it in school. But why should we have to go somewhere else? Getting that information in school would've been more helpful to me."

None of this surprises Amanda Morgan, a sexual-health educator who teaches human sexuality at UNLV. "I have students who come into my class and they don't know the proper name for their genitals. They call it a 'cookie,' a 'flower' or just 'down there.' And that's because their parents taught them it was a cookie or a flower."

A 2004 graduate of Las Vegas Academy, Morgan, twenty-six, knows firsthand what sex education in Nevada public schools is like. "I am blown away constantly by the lack of information," she says. "Students are grateful for the basic, medically accurate information they receive [in my class]. What I teach isn't based on opinion, it's based on research—this is how your body functions; this is what happens during arousal; this is how pregnancy happens."

While a few of the women I spoke with had mothers they felt they could talk to about sex, others acknowledged that if they weren't getting sex education in the classroom, they weren't going to get it at all.

"Some people can't talk to their parents about sex, so I think school is a good place to get it," Breanna says. "School is your home away from home. When I was in school, I felt my teachers were like parents. Teachers are there to help you learn and sex ed is part of that."

Veronica, who supported AB230, was surprised to learn the

bill had died. What would she say to the legislators who failed to support it?

"I would probably tell them my story, growing up not knowing anything. Not having access to basic information. Not being able to talk to your parents. I am not the only one. There are thousands of people like me."

Sharing Body Heat
Joan Price

August 2, 2008: I crawled into Robert's bed and wrapped my body around his. If I could only get close enough to make the last hour, the last months, disappear. I hugged him tightly, desperately. I wailed his name and listened to his silence, remembering his murmurs, his words of love. I nuzzled my face into his neck as I had many times before, but there was no warmth now, no "I love you, sweetheart," no kiss on the top of my head, no strong arms pulling me into him. I covered his thigh with mine, snaking my arm under his pajama top so that I could stroke the chest hair I had first touched seven years before.

I willed him to respond.

But he didn't.

I willed him to come back to life.

But he didn't.

"Do you need some time alone with your husband before the mortuary takes his body away?" the hospice nurse asked me gently. I nodded, shut the bedroom door, turned off the light, and crawled into bed with Robert's dead body.

It was the first time in three months that I could wrap myself around my beloved and hold him tightly without causing him pain. Multiple myeloma—a blood cancer that affects the bone marrow's ability to make healthy blood cells—had ripped Robert's life from him while he still lived. His fragile bones broke, causing excruciating pain. His strong dancer's body weakened and withered.

We could no longer make love—which had been our great joy—or even snuggle. Every touch was painful to him. All I could do towards the end was rest my hand or cheek lightly on his chest, or hold his hand. These little acts became making love.

Earlier that night I had held Robert's hand—the hand that painted extraordinary works of art, that gestured gracefully as he talked, that rested on the air as he danced, that caressed me for seven years. I talked to him for hours, telling him how much I loved him and recounting memories. I reminisced about the afternoons that turned into evening as we gloried in the tactile paradise of each other's bodies, the rhythm of our breath in sync. Now there was no breath at all. My tears spilled onto his hand. I lifted his hand and rubbed the wetness into my cheek. "No-o-o-o!" I wailed.

Ours had been a later-life love affair—we met when I was fifty-seven and he was sixty-four. Robert Rice (yes, his name differed from mine by one letter) was a lifelong artist and a trained dancer from the age of two. He had recently moved to my area and was looking for a place to dance. He discovered my contemporary line-dance class.

The moment he walked into the room, my postmenopause-diminished hormones went into overdrive. I met his blue eyes and fell into them. I let my eyes travel to the tuft of chest hair that peeked from the *V* of his shirt, top two buttons undone, and I yearned to unbutton it the rest of the way down. Then when he moved his hips to the music, I pictured them moving under my hands and I lost my place in the dance I was teaching. It was lust at first sight.

My crush was one-sided, though. Robert kept coming to dance class, but he seemed oblivious to my interest, though it was obvious to all the other dancers, they told me later. Robert was there for dance, not romance.

Even after we started taking walks after class at my invitation, he showed no interest in moving our relationship to the next step. So after nine months of unrequited lust, I told myself, "If you don't ask, the answer is always no."

And I propositioned him.

I can't help wondering what it would feel like to hold you without footwork, I told him in an email.

He turned me down! *I don't like to rush into things,* he explained. (Rush? Nine months?) *Let's keep getting to know each other.*

But just hours later, he emailed me again—he changed his mind! "It's been a long for these old parts," he wrote. "Maybe it's time."

We made another walking date and shared our first kiss. Our first hour of kissing. Our first week of kissing. Once unleashed, we never stopped kissing.

And we fell in love.

We were in many ways a fairy-tale couple with wrinkles, finding our great love late in life, experiencing the thrills and lust of a new romance, but with the overlay of decades of life experience and mature self-knowledge. We gloried in our passionate sexuality and the discovery of how completely two people could bond.

Through our time together, we danced—in public, in private. As long as we could dance together, we knew we'd be all right. Even after his cancer diagnosis, Robert kept dancing, taking breaks when treatments made him too sick and weak, then glorying in recapturing his physicality when he could return to the dance floor.

Until...he couldn't anymore. His pain, fatigue, and broken spine sent his dance shoes to the closet. Finally he wrote a letter to our class: *Today I began home hospice care. I will no longer be joining you in dancing. Dance with Joan, and you will be dancing with me as well.*

Seven years to the day after our first kiss, I kissed Robert for the last time and rocked his dead body to the rhythm of my sobs. I covered as much of his body as I could reach with mine. I felt his body cooling, and yet—the parts of him that my body covered became warm! I didn't know that was possible! I thought his body would chill mine, but instead, those spots under my thigh, chest, arm, and belly were warming to my touch. I marveled at the power of love—as I saw it—to warm a dead body.

The hospice nurse knocked at the bedroom door. "It's time to let them take him away," she said softly. "You won't want to watch."

I released Robert's body slowly and crawled down from the bed. I didn't look back as I left, willing the picture in my mind to be Robert's strong dancer's body, his hips in motion, his vitality, his loving gaze.

I crossed the hall to my study, closed the door, opened my laptop, and started an email to the line dancers. *Robert is free to dance with us again,* I wrote.

Being a Real-Life Accomplice
Cameryn Moore

The one call that I hated the most, over my nearly five years in phone work so far, involved a man calling in with his wife, and pressing her to get it on with me. I was so angry at him for asking me to engage her in nonconsensual activity. I felt like an accomplice. This was real life; someone on the other end was actually being coerced into participation; someone was actually being directly, psychologically abused by their partner, and I was playing along. No other call has ever made me feel even half as sleazy.

Except this guy. He's a close second.

He's a regular when I'm around; he's always so excited the first time I get given his call when I come back from tour, and pretty reliably requests me when I'm consistently around in the evenings. I have no illusions that he, like all of my "seasonal regulars," is perfectly happy with whichever other phone sex operator is handling his call when I'm not available—anyway, since my seasonal availability is self-imposed, I can hardly complain—but I am happy to hear his enthusiasm.

He fantasizes about his wife being a complete cock-hungry slut. (Side note: I kinda like it when guys fantasize about the women in their lives. I mean, in our mutual imagination they could do anything, and they're choosing their wives.) This guy's cuckolding thing is multilayered: he likes watching her be greedy, he likes the idea of fucking her after a bunch of guys (and a dog) have come in her, and his calls always culminate with a worked-up rant about how loose her cunt is when he's inside her, partly because of how many dicks she's taking and partly, that's just the way her cunt is and that's how small his dick is, relatively speaking. She's loose and he's small, and he likes to see her finally filled up, the way he wishes that she would want it.

So far, so good. He wants his wife to be a slut. I imagine, though I have no stats, that this is probably pretty common. He has talked about taking pictures of her, too. She sometimes agrees to pose, but not always. He tells her that he is just jacking off to them, but I know better. I forget that I know what he does with the pictures, because he doesn't talk about them all the time, but then he mentions them and I remember. And then I feel the sleaze settle on my skin all over again.

He posts them on a fuck-my-wife site. Guys post up shots of their partners, with or without their partners' knowledge, and revel in other guys looking at and talking dirty about their partners. On one call he gave me the link and his log-in name so I could access the site and his photo collection; we sat there for ten minutes and discussed his wife's body.

This time he mentioned that other guys sometimes posted pictures of printouts of his wife's picture with their come all over it. He also asked if my boyfriend has seen the pictures yet. Shit. I forgot that I said I might show these pictures to my lovers. Shit. I am a terrible liar. Not yet, I say, if I remember I will. Of course I will not show them. Of course I will say that I showed them, and they got so hard. And he will believe me because that is how much he wants images of his wife to be seen by strangers.

I need to remember, this could be all made up. His wife could fully approve of the way he's disseminating her naked images. She could be totally getting off alongside him, but somehow I don't think so. If his wife really doesn't know about this, I hope she finds out and rips him a new one. Hell, I hope she divorces him. In my book, this is a fully divorce-worthy offense; this is frying-pan-to-the-head territory.

As angry as I am about this betrayal, my anger is muddied a little by my witnessing it, by my complicity and implied approval. It feels a little awful. Unlike all the dead babies and hard-cocked ponies and innocent little girls WHO DON'T ACTUALLY EXIST, I think this woman does exist. I desperately hope that he's making her up, but I think she actually is alive and clueless and cooking dinner regularly for this man who loves her and fantasizes about her and has completely sacrificed her right to privacy to his satisfying wank. My job is to help him with that sacrifice.

Some days I don't like my job very much.

Oops, I Slept with Your Boyfriend
Charlie Nox

I think of myself as a woman of integrity, a lady of honor, an upstanding broad. If you had asked me when I was in high school if I'd ever sleep with a man I knew was otherwise entangled, I would have given a proud and emphatic, "No way, sister."

But as I got older, this view of relationships, among other things, got complicated. I've been married, separated, divorced, monogamous, polyamorous, celibate, and in recent years I've once in a while been the "other woman."

Don't get me wrong, I'm not going out looking to fuck guys who have girlfriends. And when someone tells me they have a girlfriend, I never pressure them to sleep with me. I don't even disregard their relationship with some sort of "I don't care if you don't care," or "She'll never know." Usually I ask them what her name is and how they met. Sometimes they show me pictures.

The few times I've found myself the mistress, we have had

deep, real, meaningful conversations about their relationships and their commitments, their heart and their body. I encourage them to honor their commitments if that feels good to them. And sometimes it does. And sometimes it doesn't.

My lovers have been in complicated relationships that are basically over but they can't break up, and they are exhausted and need the kind of nurturing that you can only get when you are getting ridden hard and kissed passionately. I've had lovers with agreements that are unclear and undefined, with no way to clarify before one of us left town. I've had lovers who were very newly and casually trying out monogamy with someone and found that our long-term friendship carried more strength, connection, healing and passion than their new quasi-relationship did. More than once I've had lovers who were separated, but not divorced, and we kept things under wraps for legal or emotional purposes.

I'm not going to tell you that I ever just get carried away and oops, something happened. Far from it. In fact, I have been known to say, "Look, if I come over to your house, it will be very hard for me to be well-behaved. I don't want us to pretend we don't know what's happening here. I don't want us to say, 'Oh my, who knew we'd end up sleeping together?'" I like men who make conscious choices, and sometimes when I give that speech, they say, "You're right, we'd better not, good night." No hard feelings there. I would always rather everyone feel right about it. I have sacrificed sex that I know I could have had because I demanded we go into it with full knowledge and intent, and they only wanted to sleep with me if it was drunk or "accidental." I don't do unconscious sex—girlfriend or not.

I trust people to navigate the decisions that work for them, and think it isn't my place to police their morals. I'm not monogamous now, but when I have been, it's been my willpower and my promises and my decision to honor my commitments that has kept me from straying. I would resent someone else trying to make me be monogamous by denying me the chance to hang out with them just because I found them attractive and interesting. The few times I've found myself with a man who has a girl-friend, it has felt like an exception, a special moment outside normal rules. On paper it looks bad, but when I check in with my gut, and listen to my body, it feels right to move forward with our sexual relationship. I know some people will adamantly dis-agree with what I'm saying here. That's okay, I think you should do what feels right in your body, and if that includes never, ever being the other man or woman, then so be it. But for me, there are times—few and far between—where my body (not my libido, but my body wisdom...my gut) says that this connection is right and good and sacred. And when that happens, I pursue it. I pursue it with clarity, consciousness and purpose. I never excuse what happened, or apologize for it either.

I'm sure some women will read this and worry about being friends with me. Up until now I've never slept with one of my friend's boyfriends. I can't imagine a situation in which that would feel right in my body. There are a whole other set of promises and agreements between me and my friends. Maybe we don't have a promise to not fuck each other's partners, but we do have promises around caring for each other and if I thought my friend would be upset, I suspect I wouldn't be turned on. But if for some reason I am there with my friend's boyfriend, and we have a crazy intense connection and sleeping with him doesn't feel wrong in my body, I might do it. I feel the need however to emphasize that despite an incredibly vivid imagination, I can't actually imagine any scenario in which this would happen.

Relationships are complicated, and emotions and promises

and sex and bodies are complicated. I don't think it's possible to make absolute rules. I know that in the messy, real rawness of life, what sounds clear in theory gets muddled in practice. I have made choices in my life counter to everything I ever thought I knew about myself. That's true not just in my relationships, but also my cancer treatment, my body, money, friendships and family.

I think it's too easy to look at the black and white of a situation and judge the morality of it. And while I don't go searching for men in relationships, I also don't pretend I feel nothing when it's not the case. I won't *try* to sleep with your boyfriend, and it's extremely unlikely, but I can't promise it won't ever happen.

Pump Dreams
Mitch Kellaway

As with all impulse buys, my gut feels how incomplete my life will be without this one. When it arrives in the mail, I eagerly tear open the packaging to reveal a dazzling pink box, covered in flowers. Bubbly lavender text dances over splashy magenta waves. Its glitz has an effect on me similar to picking up a carton of milk, only to notice that today it's set to expire. I pause, put it down, then cautiously pick it up to peer closer. The picture on the website looked decidedly more badass.

Granted, once I get over my initial aversion—*why do advertisers think this neon princess mess appeals to adults?*—the clit pump inside is indeed my hasty purchase. Sitting in my hand, it resembles a plastic toy gun, with a limp rubber nozzle extending outward. A pressure gauge sits atop it, encasing a thin needle poised to flicker past zero. My childhood self would have spent days playing made-up undercover spy games revolving around this mysterious gadget. I dig out three small glass cylinders, each about a quarter inch wider than the last. I start with the smallest, a mere inch in girth, and hesitantly unzip my pants. Sitting alone in my living room, I'm still struck with a wave of performance anxiety; a silly grin makes its way across my face.

I don't have a clitoris.

Or, rather, I used to have one. But since starting my gender transition a year ago, my relationship to it has become quite complex. Testosterone, though only adding a few centimeters of enhancement, has effectively rendered it a different organ to my consciousness. And finally living my true gender has changed my relationship to it radically. All of a sudden, I feel the intense need to *look* at it.

Not that I had ever shied away from acknowledging my nub—at least ever since I had discovered its pulsing pleasures as a teenager, hushed and feverish under my sheets. But I found little reason to search for it visually more than once, especially when I needed it most. My hands simply zoomed in to do their work, all muscle memory and flourish. My clitoris was less a place on my body than a *feeling* that coursed through me when I pressed that sweet spot right below the pubic bone. My third finger searched it out, the pad just the right size to cover it and jerkily eliminate the need to locate it almost as quickly as it arose.

Ten years past this frenzied peak of pubescent lust, testosterone gives me a reason to revisit the scene. Not only because I anticipate the growth that will creep in—but because I'm hit by the same heady waves of arousal I thought I'd left behind somewhere, along with my high school diploma. Other trans men warn me this will happen, but I expect it to be quite a bit less *auto*-erotic. I might have suspected this had I considered how alive I've become to my body's wondrous capacity to grow hair. I get a thrill whenever I run my hand over my stubbly face, my downy stomach, my furry ass. But touching isn't enough; *looking* at the dark curls gathering around my belly button or shoulders, I become momentarily transfixed. I have a lot of *moments* with myself.

I feel the same wonder when I slide down my boxers, taking advantage of an empty apartment to whip out my junk—or *dig* out, rather, since it decidedly lacks a dangle. My labia are fleshy obstacles: heavy, fuzzy curtains obscuring the main act. I awkwardly arch my back to peer downward, push my fingers apart as wide as possible, and take in the most raw, pink, sensitive spot on my increasingly sensitive body. Though it takes an effort to keep it exposed, the inconvenience fades into the background as I admire its protrusion, the strong one inch of space it claims as its own.

Over the past month, I've spent stolen moments perusing other trans men's endowments online. Never one to buy into the cultural bigger-is-better phallus myth, I surprise myself with how intensely I want to know just how big my dicklit can grow. While testosterone will certainly keep working its magic for a while longer, the man-made tactic intrigues me. And so, after a few days' wait and a somewhat discouraging first attempt, I find myself once more sitting in my favorite reading chair, half-naked and warily eyeing my new pump.

My usual first step, upon handling some unknown contraption, is to pass it to my wife with a silent, befuddled look. With a theatrical sigh, she'll figure out its inner workings, quietly pleased to exercise her handy-femme skills. She'll hand it back, triumphant, with a light laugh at my hands-on hopelessness. I'd done the same with this challenge, but soon abandoned it in her presence to try again in solitude. The aura of penis-related fragility I've sensed around other men, both trans and cis, has enveloped me. I'm not quite ready, should my efforts fall short, to endure her reassurances that I am, and always will be, enough for her. The pump conjures phantom centimeters that threaten to haunt my relationship with my manhood.

In silence, I delicately hold the smallest glass cylinder, reminding myself that within a year's time, only the largest one will be able to house my package. I screw it onto the end of the nozzle and carefully place it over my now-erect flesh. I'm heartened by how, ensconced in its see-through dome, my dick already appears magnified. My hand cautiously begins working the trigger. Though I know the process should be painless, I've nonetheless braced myself for an imagined sting. Or maybe even a sharp tug—a somewhat titillating prospect, come to think of it, for a man unable to manage a firm grip on his dick. Instead, I feel nothing.

I let out the gauge's pressure, both disappointed and relieved. But I have a creeping suspicion that, like most of my solo tries with new devices, I've missed a crucial step. I release my nub, peering closely for any signs of desired engorgement or dreaded bruising, but encounter neither. I capture it again within its glass tank, emboldened to press down harder. And…nothing.

Exasperatedly, I examine the cylinder. I'm surprised to find, along with the now-familiar musky odor that's only increased with testosterone use, a slight fog on the glass. For a moment, I deliriously imagine my dick exhaling—perhaps even sighing at being held up in the quest to embody its rightful size. Recalling an instruction video suggesting I practice first on more accessible body parts, I attach the tiny dome to one hairy thigh.

Bingo! The nozzle responds with an immediate jerk, and a circle of skin rises ever-so-slightly into the dome. When I release it, a perfectly round welt marks my success. I prepare myself to try one more time on my penis, ready to enforce the seal by pressing down and holding tightly. Firmly gripping the cylinder's base, my hand pumps the trigger. Instantly, my dick is clutched in a glassy embrace. It's a new sensation, longer than any childhood pinch I endured from my brothers and more consistent than any playful nip from a neighbor's puppy. Not to mention its location on my body, so unused to any treatment besides the wipe or the rub. Definitely tolerable, and even pleasant, if I don't shift too much. I unclip it from the nozzle, set a timer, and settle in to read a book for the next fifteen minutes. But my focus is interrupted by the captivating sight of the cylinder jutting outwards from the surrounding lips. I imagine it melding with my flesh, granting me bionic penetrative power. I study its red lumpish core, transformed by the suction from a hooded clitoris to a minuscule uncircumcised phallus.

When the timer pulls me out of my rapture, I feel as if only a moment has passed. Now accustomed to the cylinder's grip, I wish that I could keep it attached day and night, stretching erectile skin and maximizing blood flow until my dick erupts from its enclosure. But I cede to the instructions and to anatomical reality: my penis can only withstand the vacuum-locked pressure for short increments of time, increased gradually up to an hour maximum. And no matter how disciplined the practice, I can realistically strive for a modest, though meaningful, plateau: two inches in length, one and a half in girth while flaccid.

Released, my dick exhibits only the faintest swell, easily dismissible as wishful thinking. But I smile inwardly, knowing the pump's done its imperceptible work. New gaps have emerged between cells, destined to keep widening through daily stints of separation. Standing up to reinhabit my boxers, I feel as I do after my occasional attempts at exercise: eager and daunted at what my body can become if I only dedicate myself to uncovering its potential.

I return my pump to its box and carry the misty cylinder into the kitchen, where I reverently wash it and dedicate a fresh towel to its drying. For now, I let it stand proudly upright next to my sink, ensuring a lively dinnertime conversation with my wife and reminding me of its promise every time I glance over.

Prostitution Law and the Death of Whores

Laura Agustín

It doesn't matter which political direction you come from: the topics of sex work, sexual exploitation, prostitution and sex trafficking seem like a Gordian knot. As long as you listen to one set of advocates and take their evidence in good faith, you are okay. But the minute you listen to another set of advocates with different arguments and evidence, everything falls apart. The way these subjects intersect leads to untenable contradictions that make progress seem impossible. Hand-wringing and ideological free-for-alls predominate.

Twenty years ago I first asked two questions that continue to unsettle me today. The first is answerable: What does a woman who sells sex accomplish that leads to her being treated as fallen, beyond the pale, incapable of speaking for herself, discountable if she does speak, invisible as a member of society? The answer is she carries a stigma. The second question is a corollary: Why do most public conversations focus on laws and regulations aimed at controlling these stigmatized women rather than recognizing their agency? To that the answer is not so straightforward.

I am moved to make this assessment after the murder of someone I knew, Eva-Marree Kullander Smith, known as Jasmine. Killed in Sweden by an enraged ex-partner, Eva-Marree was also a victim of the social death that befalls sex workers under any name you choose to call them. Immediately after the murder, rights activists cursed the Swedish prostitution law that is promoted everywhere as best for women. My own reaction was a terrible sinking feeling as I realized how the notion of a Rescue Industry, coined during my research into the "saving" of women who sell sex, was more apt than even I had thought.

Murders of sex workers are appallingly frequent, including serial killings. In Vancouver, Robert Pickton killed as many as twenty-six between 1996 and 2001 before police cared enough to do anything about it. Gary Ridgeway, convicted of killing forty-nine women in the 1980s–'90s in the state of Washington, said, "I picked prostitutes because I thought I could kill as many of them as I wanted without getting caught." Infamous statements from police and prosecutors include the Attorney General's at Peter Sutcliffe's 1981 trial for the murder of at least thirteen women in the north of England: "Some were prostitutes, but perhaps the saddest part of this case is that some were not." He could say this because of a ubiquitous belief that the stigma attached to women who sell sex is real—that prostitutes really are different from other women.

My focus on the female is deliberate. All who propose prostitution policy are aware that men sell sex, but they are not concerned about men, who simply do not suffer the disgrace and shame that fall on women who do it.

Stigma and Disqualification

Many people have only a vague idea what the word stigma means. It can be a mark on a person's body—a physical trait, or a scarlet letter. It can result from a condition like leprosy, where the person afflicted could not avoid contagion. About his selection of victims Sutcliffe said he could tell by the way women walked whether or not they were sexually "innocent."

Stigma can also result from behaviors seen to involve choice, like using drugs. For Erving Goffman, individuals' identities are "spoiled" when stigma is revealed. Society proceeds to discredit the stigmatized—by calling them deviants or abnormal, for example. Branded with stigma, people may suffer social death—nonexistence in the eyes of society—if not physical death in gas chambers or serial killings.

In the late 1990s I wondered why a migrant group that often appeared in media reports and was well-known to me personally was absent from scholarly migration literature. I came to understand that migrant women who sell sex were disqualified as subjects of migration, in some perhaps unconscious process on the part of scholars and journal editors. Was the stigma attached to selling sex so serious that it was better not to mention these migrants at all? Or did people think that the selling of sex must transport anything written about it to another realm, such as feminism? When I submitted an article to a migration journal addressing this disqualification, "The Disappearing of a Migration Category: Women Who Sell Sex"[1], two and a half years passed before its publication, probably because the editor could locate no peer reviewers willing to deal with my ideas.

Of the many books on prostitution I read back then, most dismissed the possibility that women who sell sex can be rational, ordinary, pragmatic and autonomous. The excuses followed a pattern: The women didn't understand what they were doing because they were uneducated. They suffered from false consciousness, the failure to recognize their own oppression. They were addicted to drugs that fogged their brains. They had been seduced by pimps. They were manipulated by families. They were psychologically damaged, so their judgments were faulty. If they were migrants they belonged to unenlightened cultures that gave them no choices. They were coerced and/or forced by bad people to travel, so they weren't real migrants, and their experiences didn't count. Because they were brainwashed by their exploiters, nothing they said could be relied on. This series of disqualifications led to large lacunae in social-scientific literature and mainstream media, showing the power of a stigma that has its very own name—whore stigma. Given these women's spoiled identities, others feel called to speak for them.

Rescue Industry, Legal Regimes and Stigma

The person in a helping profession or campaign is said to embody the good in humanity—benevolence, compassion, selflessness. But helpers assume positive identities far removed from those spoiled by stigma, and benefits accrue to them: prestige and influence for all and employment and security for many. Many believe that helpers always know how to help, even when they have no personal experience of the culture or political economy they intervene in. What I noted was how, despite the large number of people dedicated to saving prostitutes, the situation for women who sell sex never improves. In "Helping Women Who Sell Sex: The Construction of Benevolent Identities"[2] I reveal the key that unlocked my understanding of the Rescue Industry.

Abolitionists talk continuously about prostitution as violence against women, set up projects to rescue sex workers and ignore the dysfunctionality of much that is conceived as "rehabilitation." Contemporary abolitionism focuses largely on the rescue of women said to be victims of trafficking, targeting the mobile and migrant women I mentioned earlier, who are now completely disappeared in a narrative of female victimhood. Although much of this goes on under a feminist banner, colonialist maternalism describes it better.

In classic abolitionism, whore stigma is considered a consequence of patriarchy, a system in which men subjugate women and divide them into the good, who are marriageable, and the bad, who are promiscuous or sell sex. If prostitution were abolished, whore stigma would disappear, it is claimed. But contemporary movements against slut-shaming, victim-blaming and rape culture clearly show how whore stigma is applied to women who do not sell sex at all, so the claim is feeble. Instead, abolitionism's aversion to prostitution probably strengthens the stigma, despite the prostitute's demotion to the status of victim rather than the transgressor she once was.

Under prohibitionism, those involved in commercial sex are criminalized, which directly reproduces stigma. In this regime, the woman who sells sex is a deliberate outlaw, which oddly at least grants her some agency.

For advocates of the decriminalization of all commercial-sex activities, the disappearance of whore stigma would occur through recognizing and normalizing the selling of sex as labor. We don't yet know how long it may take for stigma to die out in places where some forms of sex work are decriminalized and regulated: New Zealand, Australia, Germany, Holland. Given the stigma's potency in all cultures one would expect it to diminish unevenly and slowly but steadily, as happened and continues to happen with the stigma of homosexuality around the world.

Prostitution Law and National Moralities

I explained my skepticism about prostitution law at length in a 2008 academic article, "Sex and the Limits of Enlightenment: The Irrationality of Legal Regimes to Control Prostitution[3]." All prostitution laws are conceived as methods to control women who, before ideas of victimhood took hold, were understood to be powerful, dangerous figures associated with rebellion, revolt, carnival, the world upside down, spiritual power and calculated wrongdoing. Conversations about prostitution law, no matter where they take place, argue about how to manage the women: Is it better to permit them to work out of doors or limit them to closed spaces? How many lap-dancing venues should get licenses and where should they be located? In brothels, how often should women be examined for sexually transmitted infections? The rhetoric of helping and saving that surrounds laws accedes with state efforts to control and punish; the first stop for women picked up in raids on brothels or rescues of trafficking victims is a police station. Prostitution law generalizes from worst-case scenarios, which leads directly to police abuse against the majority of cases, which are not so dire.

In theory, under prohibitionism prostitutes are arrested, fined, jailed. Under abolitionism, which permits the selling of sex, a farrago of laws, bylaws and regulations give police a myriad of pretexts for harrying sex workers. Regulationism, which wants to assuage social conflict by legalizing some sex-work forms, constructs nonregulated forms as illegal (and rarely grants labor rights to workers). But eccentricities abound everywhere, making a mockery of these theoretical laws. Even Japan's wide-open, permissive sex industry prohibits "prostitution" defined as coital sex. And in recent years a hybrid law has arisen that makes paying for sex illegal while selling is permitted. Yes, it's illogical. But the contradiction is not pointless; it is there because the goal of the law is to make prostitution disappear by debilitating the market through absurd ignorance of how sex businesses work.

Discussion of prostitution law occurs in national contexts where rhetoric often harks back to essentialist notions of morality, as though in this highly travelled, hybrid-culture world it were still possible to talk about authentic national character, or as though "founding father" values must define a country for all time. One intervenor at the recent Canadian Supreme Court hearing on prostitution law argued that decriminalization would defy founding values of "the Canadian community": "that women required protection from immoral sexual activity generally and prostitution specifically" and "strong moral disapproval of prostitution itself, with a view to promoting gender equality." The national focus clashes with anti-trafficking campaigns that not only claim to use international law but sponsor imperialist interventions by Western NGOs into other countries, notably in Asia, with the United States assuming a familiar meddling role vis-à-vis Rest-of-World.

Gender Equality, State Feminism and Intolerance

Gender Equality is now routinely accepted as a worthy principle, but the term is so broad and abstract that a host of varying, contradictory and even authoritarian ideas hide behind it. Gender Equality as a social goal derives from a bourgeois feminist tradition of values about what to strive for and how to behave, particularly regarding sex and family. In this tradition, loving committed couples living with their children in nuclear families are society's ideal citizens, who should also go into debt to buy houses and get university educations, undertake lifetime "careers" and submit to elected governments. Although many of these values coincide with long-standing governmental measures to control women's sexuality and reproduction, to question them is viewed with hostility. The assumption is that national governmental status quos would be acceptable if women only had equal power within them.

Gender Equality began to be measured by the UN in 1995 on the basis of indicators in three areas: reproductive health, empowerment and the labor market. Arguments are endless about all the concepts involved, many seeing them as favoring a Western concept of "human development" that is tied to income. (How to define equality is also a vexed question.) Until a couple of years ago, the index was based on maternal mortality ratio and adolescent fertility rate (for health), share of parliamentary seats held by sex plus secondary/higher education attainment (for empowerment) and women's participation in the work force (for labor). On these indicators, which focus on a narrow range of life experiences, northern European countries score highest, which leads the world to look there for progressive ideas about Gender Equality.

These countries manifest some degree of State Feminism: the existence of government posts with a remit to promote Gender Equality. I do not know if it is inevitable, but it is certainly universal that policy promoted from such posts ends up being intolerant of diverse feminisms. State Feminists simplify complex issues through pronouncements represented as the final and correct feminist way to understand whatever matter is at hand. Although those appointed to such posts must demonstrate experience and education, they must also be known to influential social networks. Unsurprisingly, many appointed to such posts come from generations for whom feminism meant the belief that all women everywhere share an essential identity and worldview. Sometimes this manifests as extremist, fundamentalist or authoritarian feminism. Sweden is an example.

Sweden and Prostitution

The population of only nine and a half million is scattered over a large area, and even the biggest city is small. In Sweden's history, social inequality (class differences) was early targeted for obliteration; nowadays most people look and act middle-class. The mainstream is very wide, while social margins are narrow, most everyone being employed and/or supported by various government programs. Although the Swedish utopia of *Folkhemmet*—the People's Home—was never achieved, it survives as a powerful symbol and dream of consensus and peace. Most people believe the Swedish state is neutral if not actually benevolent, even if they recognize its imperfections.

After the demise of most class distinctions, inequality based on gender was targeted (racial/ethnic differences were a minor issue until recent migration increases). Prostitution became a topic of research and government publications from the 1970s onwards. By the 1990s, eradicating prostitution came to be seen as a necessary condition for the achievement of male-female equality and feasible in a small homogeneous society. The solution envisioned was to prohibit the purchase of sex, conceptualized as a male crime, while allowing the sale of sex (because women, as victims, must not be penalized). The main vehicle was not to consist of arrests and incarcerations but a simple message: In Sweden we don't want prostitution. If you are involved in buying or selling sex, abandon this harmful behavior and come join us in an equitable society.

Since the idea that prostitution is harmful has infused political life for decades, to refuse to accept such an invitation can appear misguided and perverse. To end prostitution is not seen as a fiat of feminist dictators but, like the goal to end rape, an obvious necessity. To many, prostitution also seems incomprehensibly unnecessary in a state where poverty is so little known.

These are the everyday attitudes that social workers coming into contact with Eva-Marree probably shared. We do not know the details of the custody battle she had been locked in for several years with her ex-partner. We do not know how competent either was as a parent. She recounted that social workers told her she did not understand she was harming herself by selling sex. There are no written guidelines decreeing that prostitutes may not have custody of their children, but all parents undergo evaluations, and the whore stigma could not fail to affect their judgments. For the social workers, Eva-Marree's identity was spoiled; she was discredited as a mother on psychosocial grounds. She had persisted in trying to gain mother's rights and made headway with the authorities, but her ex-partner was enraged that an escort could gain any rights and did all he could to impede her seeing them. The drawn-out custody process broke down on the day she died, since standard procedures do not allow disputing parents to meet during supervised visits with children.

In a 2010 report evaluating the law criminalizing sex-purchase, stigma is mentioned in reference to feedback they received from some sex workers:

The people who are exploited in prostitution report that criminalization has reinforced the stigma of selling sex. They explain that they have chosen to prostitute themselves and feel they are not being involuntarily exposed to anything. Although it is not illegal to sell sex they perceive themselves to be hunted by the police. They perceive themselves to be disempowered in that their actions are tolerated but their will and choice are not respected.

The report concludes that these negative effects "must be viewed as positive from the perspective that the purpose of the law is indeed to combat prostitution." To those haunted by the death of Eva-Marree, the words sound cruel, but they were written for a document attempting to evaluate the law's effects. Evaluators had been unable to produce reliable evidence of any kind of effect; an increase in stigma was at least a consequence. Has this stigma discouraged some women from selling sex who might have wanted to and some men from buying? Maybe, but it is a result no evaluation could demonstrate. The report, in its original Swedish 295 pages, is instead composed of historical background, repetitious descriptions of the project and administrative detail. Claims made later that trafficking has diminished under the law are also impossible to prove, since there are no pre-law baseline statistics to compare to.

The lesson is not that Sweden's law caused a murder or that any other law would have prevented it. Whore stigma exists everywhere under all prostitution laws. But Sweden's law can be said to have given whore stigma a new rationality for social workers and judges, the stamp of government approval for age-old prejudice. The ex-partner's fury at her becoming an escort may derive in part from his Ugandan background, but Sweden did not encourage him to view Eva-Marree more respectfully.

Some say her murder is simply another clear act of male violence and entitlement by a man who wanted her to be disqualified from seeing their children. According to that view, the law is deemed progressive because it combats male hegemony and promotes Gender Equality. This is what most infuriates advocates of sex workers' rights: that the "Swedish model" is held up as virtuous solution to all of the old problems of prostitution, in the absence of any evidence. But for those who embrace antiprostitution ideology, the presence or absence of evidence is unimportant.

When Media Are King

Media handling of these incidents reproduces stigma with

variation according to local conditions. The mainstream Swedish press did not mention that Eva-Marree was an escort, because to do so would have seemed to blame her and blacken her name. In the case of a series of murders in Ipswich, England, the media's relentless talk of prostitutes led the victims' parents to request they use the term sex workers. A number of dead women on Long Island, NY, were discussed as almost "interchangeable—lost souls who were gone, in a sense, long before they actually disappeared" (Robert Kolker, *New York Times,* 29 June 2013). A woman murdered recently near Melbourne, Australia, was called "St Kilda prostitute" rather than "sex worker" or even, simply, "woman," in a place where the concept of sex work is actually on its bumpy way to normalization. I'm talking here about the mainstream, whose articles are reproduced over and over online, hammering in the clichés.

Editors who append photos to articles on the sex industry use archetypes: women leaning into car windows, sitting on bar stools, standing amidst traffic—legs, stockings and high heels highlighted. Editors do this not because they are too lazy to find other pictures but to show, before you read a word, what the articles are really about: women whose uniform is the outward sign of an inner stain. Similarly, when writers and editors use the clichéd language of a "secret world," "dark underbelly," "stolen childhoods," "seedy streets," and "forbidden fruit," they are not simply being sensationalist but pointing to the stigma: *Here's what this news is really about—the disgusting and dangerous but also eternal and thrilling world of whores.*

Cutting the Gordian Knot

Not long ago I was invited to speak at the Dublin Anarchist Bookfair on the topic of sex work as work. The announcement on

Facebook provoked violent ranting: to have me was antifeminist, against socialism and a betrayal of anarchism. I wrote "Talking about Sex Work Without Isms"[4] to explain why I would not discuss feminist arguments in the short Dublin talk. I'm not personally interested in utopias and after twenty years in the field really only want to discuss how to improve things practically in the here and now. No prostitution law can comprehend the proliferation of businesses in today's sex industry or account for the many degrees of volition and satisfaction among workers. Sexual relations cannot be "fixed" through Gender Equality policy. If I were Alexander standing over the knot I would slice it thus: All conversations from this moment will begin from the premise that we will not all agree. We will look for a variety of solutions to suit the variety of beliefs, and we will not compete over which ideological position is best. Most important, we will assume that what all women say is what they mean.

Endnotes:

1. Agustín, Laura. "The Disappearing of a Migration Category: Migrants Who Sell Sex." *Journal of Ethnic and Migration Studies*, Volume 32, Number 1, 2006, pp. 29-47.

2. Ibid. "Helping Women Who Sell Sex: The Construction of Benevolent Identities." *Rhizomes*, Issue 10, 2005, http://www.rhizomes.net/issue10/agustin.htm.

3. Ibid. "Sex and the Limits of Enlightenment: The Irrationality of Legal Regimes to Control Prostitution." *Sexuality Research & Social Policy*, Volume 5, Issue 4, 2008, pp. 73-86.

4. Ibid. "Talking about Sex Work Without Isms" http://www.lauraagustin.com/talking-about-sex-work-without-isms-dublin-anarchist-bookfair, The Naked Anthropologist, 15 February 2013.

Fisting Day
Jiz Lee

Happy International Fisting Day!

You ready for a monster post? Well, grab your lube, lie back, and relax. It's late on Thursday night and I'm typing this at one of my favorite bars, El Rio. San Francisco felt its second earthquake today. It makes me shiver thinking about the fragility of our lives, the great divides between the Earth and our existence. And then, you know, there's fisting. Crossing my fingers that the ground below my feet withholds a mighty quake, let's get this blog going.

Not too long ago, I was chatting with Courtney Trouble about our recent film *LIVE SEX SHOW,* a fundraiser for the Center for Sex & Culture filmed during the nonprofit's annual Masturbate-a-Thon. I performed with Nina Hartley for an audience of pleasure activists. The chemistry was high with me and Nina, and we jumped into each other, and we had a grand time, and during that time, her fingers and then her whole hand went inside my cunt. And then I came for the crowd and for myself, and for my friend holding a video camera for the world to see.

At least, we hope the world could see. For as long as I've done porn, distribution companies and retailers have banned the act of fisting. It feels like it's always been this way, but that's not true. It's only been a little over a decade. Antiporn movements, in particular the administrations which coincide with them, have had a bone to pick against pornography. I advocate for consensual, ethical, and expressive erotic imagery. The act of making porn is a brave, powerful, and righteous thing. We're representing marginalized communities, taking power through creating our own images of desire. As Shine Louise Houston says, as a queer woman of color, it's especially important for her to create her own sexual images. And I completely and passionately agree. Explicitly demonstrating our pleasure shows examples of healthy sexuality that have long been denied in sex education classes. Safer sex? Check. Communication? Check. Equal gender agency, you bet. Lube? Right here.

Since 2005, I've appeared in porn for DVD distribution that I knew would not include fisting, one of my favorite sex acts. Even my very first porn scene with my lover at the time. It didn't make sense that fisting couldn't be shown, but I tossed it up to the fact that porn is marketed and driven by a lot of assumptions about what sells, what sex should look like, what the people who have sex should look like, yada, yada, yada. Basically all the reasons why I knew I was doing something important.

But wait, why is fisting so important? What do I like about it? Here're some questions I've been asked about fisting:

Why is fisting important to you?

My first experiences with hand sex, where my body took in the entire fist of a lover, happened around a time of galactic sexual exploration. I was in my early twenties and it was mind-blowing. The orgasms were intense and as I was in an open relationship, it was exciting for me to have sex with friends and teach them how to fist me, to fist others, and to really enjoy practicing sex in a safe way and to experience this with lovers of various genders and sexual orientations. It was so much fun. Fisting is about being really present and in your body, and ready for a good time.

Why do you love fisting?

What I love about fisting someone vaginally is feeling them take me in. There's a moment where the person just opens up to you. Once inside, they're so warm, wet, and every little movement you make can be felt. It's something that may take time. Fisting is something that doesn't necessarily happen right away. You put a finger in. Then two. Then three, four, and then...and sometimes after long gentle coaxing, the thumb. Sometimes lovers can try several times in sex before fisting happens. But once you've got it, it's golden! You can angle your hand for G-spot stimulation. You can find your lover's "A-spot", which is just under the cervix and some like to feel a bit of pressure there. You can carefully stroke and "jerk off" the cervix, as if it were a small, internal cock. Unlike using a strap-on or dildo, a hand can feel every motion. It's incredibly intimate and really sexy. If the chemistry and connection with my partner is strong, I can literally come from penetrating someone with my hand!

As someone who loves to receive a fist, what I enjoy about it is an unparalleled feeling of fullness. The most sensitive areas of the vagina are just within the first few inches, which is where I like to use my kegel and pelvic muscles to grip snugly around a lover's wrist, which can be compared to the girth of a medium-large dildo. Deeper inside, pressure feels good for me. I like to rock my hips against a lover's hand, or hold very still and squeeze hard, creating a game where I try to hold their hand tightly in place as they move against me. I do my kegel exercises and am pretty strong so I have a lot of control over my vaginal muscles and can make myself very tight, or, allow myself to stretch open. Or pulse between the two extremes. Combining clitoral and vaginal stimulation, the network of nerves and contracting of muscles orchestrate some of the most amazingly intense orgasms I've had.

What do you say to people who think it's dangerous or scary?

Some people think fisting is intense in a bad way—that it hurts. But anyone who loves fisting knows that it can be the most intimate and beautifully connecting experience with a lover. Or really fun in a threesome—I've held the hand, fingers locked, of a lover while the two of us have fisted a friend. I've also had both my fists inside two different lovers at the same time, while they kissed intensely. I've 69ed with fisting, and I've even fisted myself!

Fisting isn't scarier than any kind of unwelcome sexual advance. However many people don't know that much about it. We learn about sex as only being penis-vagina intercourse. But sex is so much more! We don't learn much about sexual anatomy, how to communicate with lovers, or about pleasure. In fact, when we see a fist, we may be more inclined to think of it punching someone in the face because we see images of violence more commonly and at a younger age than we do sex (e.g., cartoons show characters throwing punches and shooting guns, yet won't show even a bare breast). In *This Film Will Not Be Rated,* we see the MPAA approve violent scenes with more leniency than they do sex scenes, especially ones featuring female pleasure. So when we as a culture are more familiar with a fist being used to harm someone, it's no wonder that someone who hasn't had a healthy sex-positive education about fisting would assume it is painful. In our culture we see fists as painful weapons, while I see them as revolutionary weapons of sex-positive progress. Or, you know, the ASL symbol for the letter *E.* See? That's not so scary.

What's your experience with fisting?

Personal love of the topic aside, my work in adult film has primarily featured fisting. In fact, I fist in my films more often than I've worn a strap-on. This may come as a surprise to many DVD buyers, who would never see the act as it's been edited or angled out of the scenes, with the exception of online website content for queer porn sites. I've performed as a demo model for fisting demonstrations in adult classes such as Reid Mihalko's Iron Slut: Sex Educator Showdown! and have taught it as a guest lecturer on sex ed at colleges and universities. I was also a contributor to *The Official Book of Sex, Drugs, and Rock n Roll Lists,* where my "Top Five Songs about Fisting" was censored out of the book, due to the sensitive topic...really!

So there you go. While it's not the first time I knew fisting couldn't be shown in a hard-copy DVD, this was the first time fisting was banned by a Video on Demand (VOD) company. And here's where some background comes into play. Because: WHY is it okay to show fisting ONLINE, but not in a hard-copy DVD?

Well. Here's what I know.

DVD distributors, retailers, and porn producers are afraid to sell porn if it means they might be charged with an obscenity.

Fisting appears on the Cambria List of sex acts not allowed for inclusion in content meant for physical distribution.

From PBS:

On January 18th, 2001, Adult Video News reported on the so-called "Cambria List." Paul Cambria, a longtime attorney for the porn industry, was involved in the list's preparation. The list is controversial within the industry and interpretations differ on how it was meant to be applied. Some in the industry say it represents guidelines for the box-covers of adult videos, not for the sex acts they depict. Nevertheless, there is wide agreement that the Cambria List shows how the adult industry is seeking to be more careful, fearing a potential crackdown on pornography by the Bush Administration.

The Cambria List: Box-Cover Guidelines/Movie Production Guidelines

- Before selecting a chrome please check facial expression. Do not use any shots that depict any unhappiness or pain.
- Do not include any of the following:
- No shots with appearance of pain or degradation
- No facials (body shots are okay if shot is not nasty)
- No bukkake
- No spitting or saliva mouth to mouth
- No food used as sex object
- No peeing unless in a natural setting, e.g., field, roadside
- No coffins
- No blindfolds
- No wax dripping
- No two dicks in/near one mouth
- No shot of stretching pussy
- **No fisting**

- No squirting
- No bondage-type toys or gear unless very light
- No girls sharing same dildo (in mouth or pussy)
- Toys are okay if shot is not nasty
- No hands from two different people fingering same girl
- No male/male penetration
- No transsexuals
- No bi-sex
- No degrading dialogue, e.g., "Suck this cock, bitch" while slapping her face with a penis
- No menstruation topics
- No incest topics
- No forced sex, rape themes, etc.
- No black men/white women themes

Several things are not on this list and several things are on this list, which should never have been. I mean, WTF?!

I emailed Queerie Bradshaw, who has a legal background, and she confirmed what I expected about the legal aspects behind several porn obscenity trials when it comes to bringing visibility to marginalized sexual practices. Particularly in terms of freedom of expression. She wrote back:

It's a double-edged sword because the more a topic, scene, or act becomes mainstream, the less likely it is going to be considered obscene against the community standard. But, if you're constantly censored for fear of being prosecuted, you can't make those acts known or commonplace. I know authors that have had fisting (or the mention of sex at all even) censored out of their beautiful nonerotic literary works of art. People are afraid and the only way to stop that fear is to talk about it, but you don't know if you talk about it if you're going to be prosecuted. And that is why I totally agree with you, Jiz, that this is completely and totally a free speech censorship issue and that we need to talk about how healthy it is so people stop seeing fisting as this thing that people do to degrade and dishonor another (which is justification often for censoring anything).

Despite this go-to list, another aspect about pornography and obscenity is the Miller Test, which courts use to determine what might be obscene when there's no written rule.

The Miller test was developed in the 1973 case *Miller v. California*. It has three parts:

Whether "the average person, applying contemporary community standards," would find that the work, taken as a whole, appeals to the prurient interest,

Whether the work depicts/describes, in a patently offensive way, sexual conduct specifically defined by applicable state law,

Whether the work, taken as a whole, lacks serious literary, artistic, political, or scientific value.

The work is considered obscene only if all three conditions are satisfied.

The first points are up to the standards of the community. What community? Whatever applies! That's what makes it vague. The last one in particular is held up to whatever is reasonable to a person of the United States as a whole. The Miller Test is the reason there's more freedom of sexuality online, while less on physical goods like VHS or DVDs. While there are many areas in the United States where it is illegal to mail pornography, it's more difficult to determine online community. This is especially true for queers who have found community online. Many queers think fisting is completely normal. (If not just normal: it's amazing!)

If I had a dime for every time I've given a talk and had people give me a confused "WTF?" look when I brought up the fact that fisting was banned from DVDs—"Why? What's wrong with fisting?"—I would have enough money to pay my way into Congress and provide adequate (queer and kink friendly) education to every citizen in the U.S. so that people will understand gender, sexuality, pleasure, and consent.

So here we are.

I've fisted in much of my film and online content. In fact, I think I've fisted more times than I've ejaculated or even worn a strap-on. It's that common. While I have been somewhat unfortunately hesitant to fist on film because I know about the ban, I also have the liberation with companies who have web content because I know they won't have to edit it out. I also know that film crews can film a "soft" shot of the action if they need to. It's something I've dealt with for a while now, and because the way we consume porn is changing and going more and more to the Internet, fisting will reign.

Imagine my surprise when I learned that Courtney's film submitted for VOD was denied because of the scene. Not VOD! The Internet is supposed to be okay with fisting, because it's my community who likes to see it. That's what prompted our Fisting Day. We have to let people know more about fisting. Why it's supposedly banned, why it's awesome if they've never thought about it before. Why it's okay, even political, to love fisting.

Tell Me You Want Me.
Mollena Williams

As someone who is submissive, not only in terms of power-exchange relationships but also quite sexually submissive, I field a lot of questions about what that means.

"So, do you just, like, lie there?"

"You don't care what happens to you in bed?"

"Will you just do whatever they tell you?"

"I assume you have to be spineless to be a sub."

"Awesome. I command you to suck my dick."

Well. No, no, maybe, hell no, and after you suck mine.

One of the things that get me going on rants is the assumption that so many people make that submission is tantamount to cowering in corners, waiting to be used and abused. There is an insane amount of energy, drive, will and desire that it takes to submit successfully. And by successfully, I mean to the mutual satisfaction of all involved. Because yes, submissives and slaves and bottoms need to have their needs met, too. And for some of us, one of the hottest ways we have our needs met is by providing pleasure to others, facilitating ease in their lives.

The first connection I made with how aroused I became as a result of serving someone else was an interesting by-product of a rather passionate affair I had many years ago. Interestingly, after a rather earth-shattering first meeting with a man who had a certain...something...that wound up disabling my not insubstantial defenses, and after a rather exhilarating, dangerous, edgy, deeply erotically brutal encounter, I had an unsettling epiphany. All I wanted to do was keep him happy. Bring him coffee, get his dry cleaning, buy his cigarettes (after taking note of what brand he smoked) draw his bath, find a restaurant I thought he would enjoy...anything to have him pleased with the job I'd done. And the more I did for him, the more irresistible he found me, and the dynamic fed on itself, a sexual weather system that exploded in gorgeous thunderstorms of intense passion and lustful liaisons. And when he told me how hard he got, how much he wanted to fuck me and exactly how he was going to do it, and assured me that I was the cause of all of the delicious torments that were about to be inflicted upon my quivering, sweaty, willing flesh? Well...well.

This initial experience was enough to turn my head towards a path of submission and service that I continue to walk to this day.

When I was first exploring my submissive self, I assumed that deducing and doing whatever the dominant wanted me to do would be fulfilling enough, and I would be pleased by that and that alone. This is an ideal that some people hold holy: the selfless slave, the doting submissive who only needs the sustenance of knowing they did a good job to be satisfied. That affection, feedback, love and attention from the dominant is a "gift" that may be given at the whim of the dominant, and they are not entitled to those bits of emotional nourishment. I have learned the hard way that a diet of emotional crumbs leads to spiritual starvation. There are absolutely things I need, as a submissive, as a slave, as a human in bondage, to thrive in my desired role. And that is part of what makes me who I am. It is not just me putting everything I am on the table that makes these connections erotic and beautiful and edgy and vital.

So. What about submitting, what about service, what about taking a thorough flogging, what about menial chores, what about being useful, is sexy? Why is it eroticized? What makes it hot?

In a word? Passion.

The first time I looked into the eyes of someone who was using me with a seeming disregard for my own satisfaction, saw the heat and fire in the eyes of my lover as they took what they wanted from me and effortlessly bent me to their will, when I saw how ferociously and almost dangerously aroused they became? That passion pulled me abruptly from the realm of what I had known about sex into a new place. I was rather shocked to experience the oxymoron of feeling closer to the person who was causing me intense erotic pain than I had to previous lovers who had been gentle and circumspect in their lovemaking. This realization—that the brutal edge of passion was intensely erotic and profoundly compelling to me, drove me to question many things. My sanity, first! But then what the root of that desire was. And then to question how I could have more, and more, of that energy in my life.

As I become involved in the Leather, kink and BDSM communities, I realized that that passion came in so many more flavors than even I could have imagined. The first time I was to do a rope bondage scene, I thought it would be quite tedious. It was anything but. I wrote a bit about my love for rope and how it evolved and certainly the intense desire that my partner had to see me bound and helpless fueled my own passion.

I have had other play partners for whom a very different type of play ignites their own fires. And I have discovered that, for me, asking a new play partner "Where do you want to go today?" is the best way for me to serve them and, in turn, serve myself. It can seem an evasive technique to answer a query of "What do you want to do?" with "Well, tell me what you find hot, what draws you in, what it is that made you decide to jump into this dark world." But in fact, I learn so much. The dominant whose eyes light up as they talk about scenes where their partner is squirming in embarrassment, the top who eagerly shows off an impressive selection of canes, the switch who loves nothing more than pony play because they know what it is like from both sides of the bridle, the master who is dedicated to their path of mastery and seeks their partner, their counterpart, in whom they will manifest themselves and invest their love, time and energy...all of them are now engaging in foreplay with me. Yep, foreplay. Because I am certainly turned the hell on listening to what turns other people on. And if I am interested in playing with you, I certainly need to know what pleases you most. What gets you hot the fastest, what you think about when making yourself come...over and over...in the dead of night when you are playing the film of your darkest dirtiest hottest fantasies in the private theater of your own mind.

The passion doesn't have to be for a specific type of play in order to get me hot. Someone keenly attracted to me is more likely to pique my interest than someone who does not demonstrate an intense desire to get into my pants. If I am interacting with someone, and I don't feel a particular spark, I can promise you that I will take a second look at that person if they manage to frankly express a sincere expression of the fact that they find me desirable. The people I recall with the most passion *(and when I say "recall" I mean "masturbate furiously while recalling")* are those who were the most flagrant in their lasciviousness. From the ex-boyfriend who reveled in my fat belly and became immediately hard when I took off my shirt to the lover who agonized for several long moments trying to decide to come in my cunt or in my mouth *("Both are so, so sweet, baby, I can't decide..." he whispered)*, their expressions of lust for me were hypnotic and irresistible. Passionate lust is sexy as hell. Wanting me...wanting to do bad things to me, and telling me so, wanting to possess me, use me, consume me, with ferocity and delight is an aphrodisiac like no other.

Desire is sexy. Lust is hot. Once I know what you crave the most, when you tell me you want me, and I have absorbed some of your joy and delight in these things, in me, I have a handle on how to do what turns me on the most: be aware, open, present, aroused and rarin' to go and do what it takes to bring that fantasy to form. And I know this is true for people all over the spectrum of kink. Dominant, submissive, switch, top, bottom or just a kinky motherfucker? We ALL love feeling desirable, feeling wanted, feeling like the center of the universe for our partner. Regardless if it is for a fleeting few hours of play, a quickie in a borrowed bed or a lifetime committed relationship: bringing the rawness of passion to the fore can move a quotidian encounter into the realm of heroic hedonism that will leave an impression that will not soon fade.

The Gates
Tina Horn

"I was thirteen. My friend Annie that I was with pointed to a woman on the BART train and said, 'There's my friend's older sister. She's a dominatrix.' And I was like what's that and she led me up to this woman who was all of the things that an alternative woman in the '90s was—tall, long, lean. She was wearing all this black and leather and her hair was dyed that kind of burgundy wine-red color and she had pale skin and dark eyeliner and dark lipstick and she looked really intense. Annie asked her to tell us about her job as a dominatrix and she said I have to pee really badly right now because I have a client who likes getting pissed on a lot and I was floored. I was intrigued by this idea that you could get paid to dress up and hit people or boss them around or generally be domineering. That's something I had never considered as something that was ever going to be socially acceptable for me to do. The idea that

I could look good and get paid to do it while being bossy and pushing people around was exciting. The thirteen-year-old me thought it was awesome. The twenty-nine-year-old me thinks it's pretty awesome. Now nine years into my career, I'm getting close to being the person I wanted to be in my fantasy world when I was thirteen or nineteen."—*Davina is twenty-nine years old. She has worked as a dominatrix and manager at the Gates since she was nineteen.*

In 2013, if you are in the Bay Area and you are looking to hire a lady for any number of fetish services, the first thing that you are likely to do is to look at the listings on *ErosGuide.com*. Browsing through the thumbnails, you will see asses framed by garter belts, a lot of cleavage busting out of vinyl bustiers, and many different kinds of feminine faces staring intently back at you. Among the names of women who work independently—Lucinda Archer, Selina Raven, Colette—you will see several houses: Fantasy Makers, the English Mistress, and the Gates.

The Gates' thumbnail depicts a woman in a tight black dress shoving another woman against a Saint Andrew's cross and threatening her with a paddle. Click on it, and an ad appears with eight smaller thumbnails representing a variety of the house's current crop of women.

The ad states:

The Gates has been open continuously since 1994, in the same safe, discreet and convenient location a short twenty minutes outside of downtown San Francisco.

Our home currently offers five lavishly equipped session rooms featuring a very wide array of equipment and devices, and each room has a distinct theme and ambiance, ranging from the Rubber Executive

Dungeon—a formal and severely elegant space, to the Boudoir—a gentle and comfortable setting.

Stunning as our home and facilities are, they cannot compare to the breathtaking beauty of the women of the Gates. A brief glimpse at our website will introduce you to the physical appeal of our staff, and when you meet us in person you will be delighted by the wit, charm, creativity, grace and individuality you will discover in each of the ladies.

Here are a few of the many advantages we have to offer over others in our field:

- *We are here when it's convenient for you—open seven days a week from 10am until 10pm, available in as little as thirty minutes from the time of your call.*

- *We have a large staff body and several people available at all times, allowing you both variety in the selection of the person or people you see, as well as making ever-popular group or "party" sessions an option without hassle or delay.*

- *Our ladies are of all different experience levels, body types, ages and ethnic backgrounds, giving you the opportunity to find the exact match for your preferences.*

- *Our differently-themed rooms make it possible for you to enact your fantasy in the setting that is most exciting to you.*

- *We are very competitively priced compared to many "independents" who offer services that are virtually identical to ours.*

- *We are happy to accept credit cards.*

- *We have established an excellent reputation in the community during our over seventeen years of service due to our ongoing efforts to provide you with a safe, clean, discreet, well-equipped and, most of all, fun and fabulous place to play.*

Give us a call today to arrange your session, and we look forward to playing with you!

There is a link to a website, and a phone number to call. The Gates' site has a simple red on black design. In their pictures, the women are dressed in leather boots, latex bras, vinyl corsets, satin lingerie. Some show their faces, some show their breasts. Some emphasize their feet, some their asses, some their dominance, some their masochism. They are mostly white, slender, and in their twenties. There are a few Asian ladies, a few black ladies, and a few that are curvier than the others.

If you call the number, you will be greeted by a single word: "Hello."

In the early 1990s, while grunge music was glamorizing the darkness of the American soul, when the obscene details of the American president's sex life were international news, a barely legal young woman in Oakland, California learned that there was good money to be made dressing in leather and subjecting men to exquisite torture.

This woman who would eventually take on the name Sage Travigne was nineteen years old when her friend's godmother asked her if she knew anything about bondage.

"I had tried it with my boyfriends," she says now, "but I didn't know it was *bondage*."

The friend knew of a "playhouse" a few miles east of Oakland that employed young women to see clients for something called "fantasy and fetish exploration." Sage was unquestionably attractive and naturally bossy. The prospect of making money off those qualities was very appealing; so was the idea of quitting her job as an assistant for disabled folks, where she knew she would never get a raise. Though she didn't quite understand what this new job would entail, the style and attitude seemed compatible with her love of heavy metal and sexy shoes.

So Sage took BART out to El Cerrito and interviewed with the house's "coordinator" Lorette. She was soon installed at Fantasy Makers.

Her first client was a foot fetishist and she had absolutely no idea what to do with him, but after a few sessions she began to realize she was a natural. The work suited her. The way Fantasy Makers was run, however, did not. Nothing was designed in a way that made Sage feel sexy, and she didn't like the way Lorette condescended to her.

Eventually she moved to another house called the Shadows, which had classier facilities but presented other problems. The owner of the Shadows was male, and he shamelessly slept with his employees. Sage found it equally offensive that he charged the working ladies for sodas and snacks.

After nearly two years of working for others, Sage decided she had learned enough about clients to run her own operation. She rented a small apartment on Woolsey Street in Berkeley and took out an ad in *Spectator* magazine. She got male friends to do security. Eventually she had so many clients trying to book her, she began to wish she could be in two places at once. That led to her inviting other female friends to take sessions out of her space. As she realized she was running an organization, she decided to give it a name with an appropriate mystique: the Gates.

The early days of the Gates were a lot of fun for dommes and clients alike, but the whole thing would have certainly collapsed after a few exciting months if it wasn't for Sage's natural talent for order and accountability.

"Every rule at the Gates is based on a reaction to something that I didn't like about other people I worked for," she says.

Business continued to improve, so much that she was able to afford renting a much bigger house in Oakland. This place, which she now calls The First Big House, had enough space that she and her then-boyfriend Mark could build unique wooden bondage structures. With the extra money that was coming in she invested in more furniture, nicer gear, and bigger ads.

In January 2006, Sage was able to afford to move to a larger house across the street. She now employed around twenty women. At mandatory monthly meetings, they addressed interpersonal conflicts, and collectively brainstormed how the house could run more effectively.

At the first meeting after acquiring the New Big House, Sage said, "Well, ladies, the good news is, we're not having a meeting tonight!"

There were cheers. The only thing a collective loves more than a meeting is no meeting.

"The bad news is, we're moving!"

There were groans.

So in the early winter evening, twenty-some plainclothes dominatrices hauled boxes marked Executive and Blue Room and filled with leather, rubber, wood, metal, and linens across 57th street to the new Big House, where the Gates has operated ever since.

In cutoff jean shorts and cotton tank tops, Sage is every bit the California golden girl. She has a slender, athletic build, with breasts and hips large enough to be vivacious without being "curvy," and a clear, tanned face. Her hair is auburn-colored, and her eyes are icy blue. She is vegetarian, and fond of Newcastle beer. Even when she is being silly, which is often, she possesses an unwavering solemnity. When she puts together an outfit from her stunning closet of fetish gear, that calm demeanor, along with tight rubber corsets and six-inch black stilettos, holds her body high and proud.

Nowadays it would be an understatement to describe Sage as

someone who understands bondage. At the age of thirty-nine she has been managing the Gates for nearly twenty years. Of all the kinky things she has learned to do, tying people up remains her favorite. She has grown from an opportunistic teenager with a penchant for thigh-high boots to one of the Bay Area BDSM scene's most established bosses.

Though she no longer takes sessions, Sage continues to teach the difference between a square knot and a granny knot to countless young women who are curious, as she once was, about this particular kind of sex work, and who want to learn about it in a woman-friendly environment.

In 2006, I was one such woman. I worked for Sage first on staff and later as a "right-hand man" manager, for four years. No other experience has changed my life so profoundly for the better.

It's 9:30 a.m. on a Wednesday in mid-June and the morning shift is arriving at Oakland's premier house of BDSM.

In a sense, "The Big House"—as it's known to the ladies who work there—is the actual two-story Victorian house, which— due to careful soundproofing and window boarding—blends in with the other homes in its working-class neighborhood. "The Gates" is more of an abstract place, a state of mind. It is, as the name implies, a threshold. Through this opening, you may, for the price of admission, enter a world in which it is possible for your erotic fantasies to become real.

Some employees arrive by car, some by bicycle. Some walk from the nearby BART station. Some women's partners drop them off, and some spring for cabs. Sage is a dog owner, and allows her workers to bring theirs to work, so there is usually a motley pack lounging behind the tall wooden fence of the backyard.

The coworkers greet one another enthusiastically. Morale is

high. Autumn, who has long, straight, brown hair and a bombshell figure poured into a white velvet tracksuit, is the manager today. She grabs a clipboard off a nail in the kitchen wall and begins to assign tasks.

"Celio, can you do inventory? Louise, I know you like to sweep. I'll take care of the recycling and the rubber wall polishing."

After greeting her employees, Sage settles herself at her office desk with a meticulously organized datebook and a pint glass of steaming herbal tea.

The other women, who range in age from precocious eighteen to a very well-preserved forty-year-old, get straight to work without complaining. If there is a prima donna among them she does not take this moment to reveal herself. Dishes are put away and the whistling kettle is taken off the stove. Yards of cotton rope are pulled out of the dryer and coiled. When the chores are done, the women settle down at the kitchen table with black coffee and bottles of kombucha to discuss, along with their outrageous sexual exploits, life's more mundane subjects—television, children, car trouble.

These routines are the only action in the house for about half an hour. Then, the phone rings.

The answering tension emanating from the ladies in the kitchen is palpable through the entire house. They have been trained to answer the phone before the fourth ring, and to put aside anything they might be doing—cooking breakfast, painting nails, doing homework—to prioritize the phone. On the other end of the line is the potential for money. And, regardless of their individual motivations, money is what they're all here for.

This is a business, after all.

"Hello," Sage says, in a voice just a few registers below her usual speaking tone. She doesn't say, "Thank you for calling the Gates," or "This is Sage," or "How can I help you?" Her phone voice has a cool, emotionless femme-fatale quality. It's not the accommodating voice of a perky secretary or the alluring voice of a phone-sex operator. Sage means business on the phone. She does not believe in flirting to get clients to book. She doesn't "give free phone sessions."

Sage asks the client what he's interested in. She keeps the conversation focused on availability, times, and other practical concerns. When he arrives, the client will have a chance to discuss more intimate details with the woman he books.

The price starts at $160 for an hour, and is referred to as a "Donation." It is nonnegotiable. The rate increases, with up-sell craftiness, to $220 for ninety minutes, $280 for two hours, and so on through overnight sessions. Adding a second lady to your scene costs an extra hundred an hour. Adding a lady for a "walk-on" or cameo appearance is $20 for ten minutes, $40 for twenty, $50 for a half an hour. Bringing another lady in for a golden shower is $20 even if it takes less than ten minutes.

Some people call the Gates because they have a very specific fantasy they can't get off their mind. Many imagine that if the fantasy is consummated it will lose its obsessive hold. Sometimes this works and sometimes it doesn't.

Some clients are hobbyists. For them spanking is like tennis and bondage is like cooking class. These people consider themselves connoisseurs of an experience, and of the professional ladies themselves.

Some clients are enchanted by the general idea of dark, cruel women, of non-normal sexuality. Some of these people have no idea what they're getting themselves into.

Some clients are looking for a mistress for an ongoing professional relationship, the way that other people might search for a good stylist, personal trainer, or therapist.

Some clients want to lie on their back while a woman literally walks all over them. Some of them want pedicured feet, or piss, or a silicone dildo in their mouths. Some want to be locked in a closet and ignored. Some want to be completely mummified in Saran Wrap. Some want the surface of their skin pierced with 24-gauge needles. Some want a gallon of water sprayed up their rectum with a shower nozzle. Some want a key-lime pie in the face. Some want to be called slave, slut, dog, whore, toy, butt-boy, worm, scum, or pathetic worthless cum dumpster.

Some arrive with scripts, with duffle bags of personal toys, with outfits for themselves, with outfits for their mistress.

Some want somebody to talk to.

When you book a session at the Gates, you arrive right on time. You ring the bell, and step through the front door to a glass-walled porch filled with potted houseplants. The door to the house swings open, and you enter.

Behind the door stands the lady you've booked your session with. She ushers you into a living room and sits you down on an enormous, comfortable, black leather couch. On the coffee table before you are some large hardcover books of fetish photographers Erik Kroll and Doris Kloster. To your left, freshwater fish swim in an enormous tank.

Your mistress sits opposite you on another, smaller couch. She may be in a dress, or robe, but she is not naked or in fetish gear. One of the rules of the house is that negotiation is conducted between two consenting adults with as little distraction as possible. Regardless of whatever depraved roles you may eventually play, this is a professional discussion.

She smiles, and greets you with pleasantries, like an old friend or a hairdresser. Then she gets down to business. What are you in the mood for today? What's your fantasy? What are your turn-ons? What are you curious about, and what is an absolutely boundary? Do you have specific attire requests? Are you interested in a walk-on from another lady? There may be a new girl in training: how would you feel about her sitting in on the session?

She might ask you about any safety concerns you have. Can you be on your knees for long periods of time? How's your heart?

She suggests you "get business out of the way," and you hand her a bank envelope, or a gift bag, or a sweaty wad of bills. She retreats with a smile behind a thick black curtain to an unseen room. For a few minutes you wait, wring your hands, stare at the fish, flip through an art book. Your heart pumps and your imagination runs wild.

Behind the curtain is the world you don't see.

Sometimes the woman who walks through that curtain becomes another person when she's not putting on a show for you. The glamour melts away, replaced by conspiratorial winks, or weariness. Sometimes the woman is the same whether she is arriving, sweeping the floors, or flogging a naked man.

There are people who would probably pay good money just to be chained up so they could silently observe this backstage area: the office, the kitchen, the locker room basement, the back porch. But that is not on the menu. Though countless scenes can be created within these walls, the world on the other side of the door is one to which no amount of money can permit you access.

Presently, your mistress returns, and probably says something commanding like, "Follow me," or something cute like, "Right this way to your doom!"

You can learn a lot about someone based on how they react to the news that you're working as a professional dominatrix. Upon learning that I loved this mysterious work, my old friend Lucas mused, "If I had the money to go to that house, I'd hire all the girls for the night and we'd all get naked and just do something totally ordinary...like order a pizza!"

My mother asked, "What's a dominatrix?"

And my friend Jason said: "Good. You're going to learn a lot about men."

What Jason had wrong is that being a sex worker merely confirmed everything I already knew quite well about men. Clients, with all their wildly diverse ages, classes, ethnicities, values, manners, and desires, have always been a snap for me.

What I never expected to learn through working in a bondage house was how to love women.

Sage created something I had never been a part of before: a place where powerful women supported one another to get the project of making money done safely and efficiently. The Gates is a rare business in which all the workers are female and—with one or two notable exceptions—all the customers are male.

While we were working at the Gates, we weren't only powerful because we were the ones holding the ropes and the whips (although that literalization of dynamics certainly helps drive the point home). We were powerful because we were women who guided men into sexual discovery. Both clients and workers learned things about themselves in session, but it was the females who were the guardians of the mystique.

Men entered, and made themselves more vulnerable to strangers than they did to anyone else in their lives. Then they left, all without knowing the first thing about how the house was run. For the most part, they were like fine diners who arrive at a restaurant without ever considering what goes on in the kitchen. Certainly, some clients thought we all just materialized, corsets cinched, as soon as they wanted us. That we were never tired, or feeling unsexy. That we never got colds.

The truth, of course, is that someone was always rushing to lace up her boots, and someone was always complaining about her numbers, and sometimes we just sat around all afternoon, waiting for the phone to ring.

We all had different motivations for being there, and we didn't always all see eye to eye. But there was a reason we all worked in a house instead of going solo. When a girl went into session, she knew she wasn't alone.

Because whether she'd had five Steves that day or only one half-hour golden shower or whether she'd been sling height and elbow deep in a middle-aged man or been rubbed down in baby oil, whether he'd respected her dignity or she'd spent two hours batting greedy hands away, whether she felt very powerful or very small, whether she'd forgotten her troubles or been reminded of them, whether she'd been a schoolgirl or a satanic nun or a cuckolding wife, whether she'd been pretending not to watch the clock, or finding herself being strangely turned on by creepy "Uncle Mike" who talks like Jack Nicholson—she could kick off her stilettos and unzip her leather and collapse in laughter or burst into tears. She knew that these women, whether in sweats or cocktail dresses or lacy panties or nothing at all were there for her—to break the spell, to help her stain another coffee mug or champagne flute with red lip prints, to commiserate and corroborate and remind her she was real.

What struck me most about working for Sage was how much it reminded me of my best experiences with cooperative living. The decency of the house's rules made it possible for women to make good money working outside of established commercial systems that often oppress them or limit their options. And the careful attention to safety concerns made it possible for clients to have experiences that were dangerous in more abstract realms of the psyche.

In my time there, I learned enormous amounts of practical kink skills like bondage tricks and the proper way to choke someone out. I also learned profound things about the human sexual imagination. The most important of these is the role that irony plays in fantasy: the dark, depraved, degrading scenes that are commissioned around the clock at the Gates are predicated on respect and clear communication. The implied meaning of a scene is most often the opposite of the literal meaning.

At the Gates, sex is dressed up in darkness, but I have never been around so many giggles, so much emotional catharsis, so much evident healing.

When playing at the Gates, you have five choices of environment. Across from the negotiation room is the Executive Dungeon. Here, the ceiling is painted a muted gold. The walls are made of black rubber. On one wall is a wooden Saint Andrew's cross, and in the corner is a leather-upholstered spanking bench. In the center of the space is the house's most impressive and unique piece of furniture. A stainless-steel bed with hooks all up and down its four posters. This room is elegant, understated despite its scandalous setting. A wooden suspension bar hangs from a rig in the ceiling. Every room, in fact, has one of these rigs, and each one can support a three-hundred-pound man.

The boudoir is next door. Painted a lively green, it contains a matching white IKEA bed, vanity, and wardrobe. Inside the wardrobe are size-13 high-heeled shoes, enormous panties, panty hose, and costume makeup. This room is suitable for domestic scenes, cross-dressing, or sensual sessions that involve oral worship of a lady's feet, legs, ass, or breasts (never, it must be emphasized, her vagina or anus, and it is extremely rare for a lady to kiss on the mouth). It also attracts clients who have physical limitations and need to spend most of the session sitting or lying down.

Through the foyer and up the hardwood stairs is the house's top floor. The office/schoolroom is first. In it is a wooden desk large enough for a small person to lie flat on his or her stomach, a small linen couch, and—somewhat incongruously for the setting—another leather spanking bench. Role-plays involving school or work or doctor's offices are very common, because these are primal places for power dynamics to manifest.

Next is the Blue Room or Worship Room, in which there is another wooden cross, a man-sized cage with a leather table for a top, and a closet converted into an iron jail cell. The midnight blue of the walls and numerous mirrors makes the place seem much more cavernous than its true dimensions.

Lastly, the red room is draped floor to ceiling in red curtains that evoke the nightmare scenes of "Twin Peaks." A wooden structure designed for all kinds of bondage dominates the space, though somehow there is also room for a leather futon and wooden riding horse with real equestrian saddle. There is a warmly erotic Parisian boudoir feeling to this space.

Every room contains the following items: a spray bottle of Madacide (medical-grade disinfectant), water-based lubricant, at least ten condoms, several carabineers, some kind of bondage cuffs, several coils of cotton rope, at least one flogger, a Wartenberg wheel, a blindfold, a collar, a leash, metal nipple clamps, a collection of clothespins, tea light candles and votives, a box of matches, and an assortment of intimidating dildos.

The other doors on the second floor lead to: a linen-supply closet filled with lube, towels, sheets, and enema bags; the bathroom, which contains a bathtub for golden and brown showers (the only room in the house with a window that isn't frosted or boarded over); and, the upstairs apartment where Sage used to live. Trusted friends inhabit the apartment; it is the only space in the entire house that is not designated as the Gates. A stereo blasts punk music in that apartment all day to muffle the sounds of mundane life: someone in the Red Room can hear everything that goes on in that apartment, and vice versa.

Regardless of which room you chose, what happens when you enter is between you and your mistress.

Only once did I ever make the mistake of trying to spend the night alone at the Gates.

I was living in San Francisco and commuting to the East Bay every weekend to work the Friday evening and Saturday morning shifts. This was right before the 2008 recession, and my business was unbelievable. I saw four to five clients a day on average. In the space of eight hours or so I easily did more sexual experimentation than most humans will do in a lifetime.

On these shifts, I worked myself up into ecstatic states of concentration and adrenaline, and completely forgot that the rest of the world with its formalities of politeness even existed. Fueled by pure fantasy, I rarely had time to eat. About twenty minutes after closing the door on my final client of the day, I was always struck by a ravenous need for the macaroni and cheese we kept stocked in bulk next to boxes of Small, Medium, and Large latex gloves. I would shovel food into my face like a teenage athlete, and still continue to lose weight. Yeah, I was in it for the excellent money, but I had never before experienced such a concentrated dose of the human condition. For a perpetually curious person such as myself, it was a dream job.

Usually I spent the night between shifts with friends in Oakland, but this particular Friday I had a very late client and another one scheduled for first thing the following morning. I figured it would just be easier to sleep on the bed in the Executive.

By this point, the Big House felt like my second home. Sage encouraged us to greet arriving clients the way a hostess would treat distinguished guests. When I showed up for my shift I would stash my bike in the basement and immediately tear off all my clothes—my sweatshirt, cotton leggings, sneakers, men's boxer briefs, sports bra, band T-shirt. In fact I was quite notorious among the ladies for conducting my "behind the scenes" affairs—vacuuming, organizing the datebook, counting my money, doing paperwork—in the buff.

The Gates gave me permission to toss out any shame or confusion I had about my body and feel like a sexy woman who had no need for social niceties like clothing. Subsequently I have rented other dungeon studios where the owners are shocked by my immodesty. More than once it has been necessary for me to sheepishly explain that dungeons and nudity have become synonymous in my mind.

It was in this relaxed and naked state that I locked the door behind the last ladies working late on the Friday night shift, and settled into the Executive bed. I am quite proud of my ability to make a home anywhere I lay my head, and I never considered that the Big House would be any different.

That night I discovered that the wrought-iron bed in the Executive Room was not made for sleeping.

Maybe stagehands have similar experiences if they get caught working late at the theater and must spend the night in a prop bed on a stage. In my dreams, every scene that had ever taken place in that room seemed to be happening at once. All night I tossed and turned as if I were trying to sleep in the middle of a kinky symphonic light show. Surreal moments of nipples extending and whips raising welts flashed through my mind. All sort of obscenities were barked over each other, as if every booth at a porn shop were turned up at once.

These ghosts of the Gates were not nightmarish per se. They were just dreams that were meant for waking life, not for quotidian human functions like resting. The house Sage built had spawned a million spontaneous stories, and those stories, once given a life of their own, had entered my psychically vulnerable subconscious. They were more powerful than either the men or women who'd first conjured them during working hours; now, without the other women to protect me, I was defenseless against them.

I never slept there again, and I recommended that other girls refrain from doing so as well. But I had a new reverence for the power of the place.

Sage does not take sessions anymore. In fact, she stopped around the time I started. I was fortunate enough to see her in action once or twice when someone wanted a walk-on and no other lady was around. On one such occasion, I clomped out of the session bathroom to find Sage drinking an afternoon beer in her office.

"I need someone for a golden shower walk-on!"

Sage looked at the books and shrugged. "Well, I guess it's gonna have to be me."

"Is that okay?"

"Sure thing, Mistress. I'll see you up there," she said, and tipped the rest of the beer down her throat.

In five minutes, just as I was finishing pissing, there was a knock on the door. My client—lying in the bathtub as all toilet-training submissives did—spluttered, "Come in!"

Sage entered the tiny bathroom. She was wearing a transparent blue teddy and no makeup, her blonde-red hair and sun-tanned skin radiating beauty.

"Well, look at this boy," she cooed. "It looks like he hasn't quite been doused enough."

Moving gracefully, like a barefoot ballerina, she mounted the lip of the tub and released a steady stream of hot piss all over the client, who may not have even realized how lucky he was.

The Choice of Motherhood
and Insidious Drugstore Signage
Stoya

I had the privilege of growing up with a second wave feminist/ reformed hippy mother. Before I sprouted my first pubic hair she handed me a mirror and a flashlight and told me to get to know my vagina. I was raised to believe that my body was mine to share with whoever I chose, whether that was one man, a couple of women, or a whole bunch of people over the course of my life. My mom homeschooled me for most of my childhood, and the parts of history that most excited her were the struggles for social change. When I was in fourth grade we drove down to Atlanta and took a tour of an old plantation. Afterwards we stood on the giant lawn and my mother's bright green eyes turned an unsettling shade of yellow from emotional overstimulation as she educated me about the history of -isms in America and how important freedom and tolerance are.

A year or so later we found this book, *The Movers and Shakers,* in a used bookstore outside of Charlotte. It was about activists in the sixties. The black cover with orange and yellow writing made the contents seem urgent but the dust and used-book smell made it seem old and historical, like something important had happened in the distant past. This book prompted my mother to share her own experiences of being a young adult in the early seventies. She'd fought for civil rights, she'd celebrated when *Roe v. Wade* was decided in favor of reproductive rights, and she'd been the only woman working in the engineering department at a nuclear plant when she got pregnant with me. I was ten or eleven when I first heard these stories. I thought my mom was positively ancient and I had little contact with other kids or the outside world. I believed she'd helped make the world a better place a very long time ago and thought that everyone was accepting of everyone else now. I thought that all the battles for human rights had been won already and I imagined prejudice as a relic of the past; if it still existed it must have been decaying next to a gramophone or icebox in a junkyard somewhere. I saw the effects of the sexual revolution and the right to abortion as gifts that my mother's generation had given mine.

The first time someone tried to shame me for sexual activities, I thought they were the cultural equivalent of the missing link. It took me years to really understand that there are at least as many anti-equality, anti-sex work, anti-homosexual, and anti-all sorts of other things people in the world as there are people who think like me. Sometimes I still forget. For instance, when I said in my first article for *Vice* that "I've been pretty successful at avoiding pregnancy," I was surprised when people assumed that meant I'd never had an abortion. What I should have said was that given the amount of sex I've had (and without doing the actual math) three abortions seems statistically low. In the same way I feel entitled to have the kind of sex I want to have, purchase condoms, leave the kitchen, wear shoes, and put my body through attempts to find a hormonal birth control method that works for me, I feel entitled to have an abortion when necessary. They're a last resort and I do try to avoid them, but an abortion is still a better option in my opinion than an unwanted child. All three of my abortions were medication induced. Taking RU-486 to end a pregnancy is more painful than my worst period but less painful than a burst ovarian cyst.

Just like I prefer to avoid getting pregnant at all, I'd prefer to always catch unwanted pregnancies as early as possible and avoid the more invasive aspiration or dilation and evacuation procedures. I will take a pregnancy test if I don't see my period for twenty-nine days or if it's suspiciously light. I've been on Loestrin 24Fe (a kind of hormonal birth control) since January 7th. I take my pill every single day between 7:00 and 9:00 a.m. I missed one of the placebo/iron supplement pills about a month ago and took a double dose the next day. I've heard that this pill occasionally causes women to stop menstruating entirely, but I haven't seen anything resembling full-on menstruation for a suspiciously long time and I have actually taken pregnancy tests when I haven't even touched a penis for months just to see the little minus sign or the "not pregnant" and be happy that there's at least one thing that isn't currently a problem if I'm having a bad week. So I went to the drugstore a couple of days ago and got a pregnancy test from the family planning aisle.

The phrase family planning hanging on a sign above the pregnancy tests and condoms irritates me because it implies that everyone plans to have a family at some point. As the cashier was ringing me up another woman behind the counter asked me how my day was going. I told her that I was on birth control, pointed out that I was purchasing a pregnancy test and a bottle of Aleve, and said she probably didn't want to hear the actual answer. She chuckled awkwardly and wandered off. I usually go for EPT or Clearblue, but this time I went with First Response. When I pulled out the test and instructions, a cardboard gizmo fell out. First Response has taken the presumption that everyone wants to have a baby one step further by including a congratulatory contraption that tracks one's due date and has a helpful form on the back for "Moments & Milestones" including possible baby names, birth time, and weight. I'd hoped that the asterisk next to "A general guide for your enjoyment" would lead to a footnote saying "You know, if you're interested in having a baby." But it was a disclaimer stating that only a physician can determine due dates. I grumbled while I waited three minutes for the results and seethed when both tests came up with error messages.

Inferior products aside, the thing that makes me angry is the insidious suggestion that all women want children and the subtle shaming of people who exercise their reproductive rights. This is part of the reason women feel the need to say things like "I only had one abortion" or "a baby at that point would have ruined my college prospects." I resent the way this sneaky societal pressure has wormed itself into my brain enough that I feel the need to explain my mild latex allergies and issues with hormonal birth control or follow the number of pregnancies I've terminated with a reminder of how many sexual acts I've engaged in when talking about my own abortions. I'm uncomfortable about the way that I've allowed these messages to undermine my belief in my rights enough to feel defensive about exercising them. Every time that a woman like Molly Crabapple or Chelsea G. Summers vocally stands behind their decision to abort, it's a drop in the bucket that maintains balance against people like Todd Akin and Jack

Dalrymple. It reminds me that the freedoms we do have are precarious and that a sizable chunk of America sees women, homosexuals, and anyone who is different than they are as lesser beings.

And it makes me that much more appreciative of those who do support freedom of choice.

Kinky, Sober and Free: BDSM in Recovery
Rachel Kramer Bussel

What's the link between BDSM—the catchall term for bondage, discipline, domination/submission, sadism and masochism—and sobriety?

Can you be clean and sober and still engage kinkily? For those who identify as clean and kink-friendly, the answer is a resounding, "Yes, please (may I have another?)." The connection is being borne out as supportive communities of like-minded people are springing up around the country.

The issue goes beyond physical safety; as one woman told me, "Who wants to be flogged by a drunk guy?" While a number of interviewees reported they have attended play parties—often in private homes—where alcohol and drugs abound, most organized play parties frown on, or explicitly forbid, such substances and often turn away players who show up intoxicated. (This is also a common complaint of professional dominatrices, who often have to turn away drunks.)

Mollena Williams—a BDSM educator and the coauthor of the guidebook *Playing Well with Others*—founded San Francisco's Safeword, which offers a "12-Step modeled approach to recovery for kink-identified people." She began the group in 2007 in response to her lukewarm reception at traditional AA meetings. She recalled that her tastes were considered to be incompatible with her sobriety: "People are often ready to attribute your desires to do kink or BDSM as part of your addiction." She added that many 12-steppers "equated that high you experience within a scene as a result of a dry drunk. I was accused of substituting one drink for another. They didn't see that for me Kink and Leather were the last bastions of my sobriety!"

The majority of interviewees emphasized the positive effect BDSM has had on their sobriety, going far beyond the realm of the dungeon or kinky world. Theener, a thirty-five-year-old New Yorker who's been kinky since she got a birthday spanking in 2004, feels like she had to "learn how to be kinky all over again" after getting sober in 2008.

"You have to learn how to have fun without alcohol and drugs being the center of your fun," she said. "When I wasn't sober, I wasn't interested in spaces like [S&M club] Paddles and [support and information group] Lesbian Sex Mafia meetings because there wasn't booze. I had to appreciate later that those places were alcohol free."

Theener makes an explicit link between how BDSM and sobriety work together in her life. "I describe myself as having a dopamine problem; one of the things that's been integral with me in sobriety is figuring out healthy ways to experience adrenaline-creating activities," she said. "BDSM is a way that I can get all the chemicals in my brain revving and it keeps me busy and learning. It's somewhat risky but because it's surrounded on all sides by boundaries and negotiations, it's a safe way of engaging in some risky behavior that's helpful in my sobriety."

Jonathan, thirty-five, of Brooklyn, got into kink after sobering up. He found that exploring BDSM "dovetailed nicely" with a 12-step program. "The thing that surprised me and made me really happy when I started to explore this world is how healthy and sane the people are," he said. "From the outside you'd think BDSM freaks would be damaged misfit toys—and there are those people—but there's also a community of people who are very aware of who they are, very aware of the boundaries and of the consequences of their actions."

Similarly, Jackson, thirty-six, of San Francisco, sought out the kink scene specifically as a way of coping with sobriety. "Part of my motivation for exploring play parties is because after I lost my favorite means for medicating my social anxiety, it became much more difficult to navigate daily, run-of-the-mill interactions," he said. "I figured the one place where everyone would be both open-minded and accepting of awkwardness would be a pansexual play party space. It offers a respite from shame, guilt and judgment. The party I frequent, Mission Control, is not a sober space, but I'm comfortable around alcohol at bars so it isn't a problem."

As BDSM has become more and more mainstream over the years, the resources for sober kink have also increased. The kink-centric networking site FetLife has a "clean and sober pervs discussion group" where posters can seek local sponsors, list sobriety dates and, of course, hook up. Recovery in the Lifestyle is a fellowship of BDSM lifestyle people who are in recovery—or would like to be—and serves as a hub for those looking to find meetings or start them. Kink Aware Professionals List, put out by the National Coalition for Sexual Freedom, is a directory that can provide you with a kink-friendly therapist. Even Princeton University's newly formed BDSM/kink support group PINS (Princeton in the Nation's Service) has a strict no-alcohol policy. And if you are put off by the style of *Fifty Shades of Grey*, *Kinked Sober* is a terrific—and free—*Story of O*-type e-book with a sober twist, by the very anonymous-sounding Lauren L.

Practitioners still have to be wary, however. "The flip side," warned Jonathan, "is that a lot of people in recovery have also had problems with sex addiction. Any substance or behavior can be abused. If you want to explore your desires, how do you do it in a way that is healthy and doesn't start to tip into compulsive behavior?"

Williams proclaimed that kinky and sober people are "fortunate" in another respect. Alcohol and drugs are "pretty much a nonissue in the majority of BDSM spaces, in contrast to the time when bars were the primary meeting place for the leather community. Kink space is, more often than not, sober space." Given that sensory play offers its own high, she insists, alcohol and drugs become less relevant. She added that many of the kink, leather and BDSM conferences "even have their own recovery meetings slated into the event schedule, and if they don't, will usually give up free space for such gatherings."

Theener found one such meeting on the agenda at South Plains Leatherfest, an annual Dallas weekend event, and calls it one of the best meetings she's ever attended. "I had no idea there was going to be sober support there at all, and I was pleasantly surprised to find a 12-step meeting on the agenda," she said. She had been planning to seek out an outside meeting, so this space was especially welcoming.

Others have had differing experiences. Paola, thirty-five, of New York, who's been openly kinky since 2005 and sober since

2006, is partnered with another sober kinky person, but hasn't found the scene as welcoming. "I wouldn't say the BDSM world is not supportive to sober kinksters. I just think that the BDSM world doesn't go out of its way to think of events for us or to keep us in mind when planning. Most of the sober kink events are boring and unimaginative. It seems like in the kinky world a sober space / event is synonymous with 'not any fun.'"

For Paola, this lack of fun was not about danger so much as the lack of action. "Workshops!" she declared. "I love learning, but after a while you want to get together to play." She cited events and spaces such as Paddles in New York. "I love that this space is available," she said, "but it has to be one of the cheesiest and most boring BDSM venues in the city. The price is just not worth going there to play. The fun events there tend to be private ones that do have alcohol." Ouch.

For those thinking of exploring BDSM, before jumping head-first into play parties, Theener recommends attending casual, nonsexual gatherings called "munches," where "you can meet up with people in their normal clothes at a diner and everybody can get to know each other. It's a low-pressure environment and re-minds me of fellowship after an AA meeting." Look up your city and "BDSM munch" to find one near you.

If you decide you are ready to negotiate some play, "Justine," an anonymous twenty-eight-year-old San Franciscan who's been sober since 2006 and involved in BDSM since 2008, offers some hard-won advice: "If you are negotiating play with someone, be sure to specifically bring up intoxicant use. While it is generally frowned upon in the wider kink scene to engage in SM while totally inebriated, many people do participate in various forms of kink while using, and one cannot assume anything about a potential partner's habits."

Paola's advice for newbies? "Ask a lot of questions! You may think a potential play partner is sober but they may have a different definition. I've experienced folks who are 'sober' but still smoke pot or do ecstasy. Be very clear about any parties you go to and what drugs/alcohol will be there. A lot of people assume you will be fine playing with inebriated folks. Stand up for yourself and be clear that is not what you are looking for."

Williams warned, "Be aware that there are some places where alcohol is a central feature to the play. Some fetish nights are so booze fueled, it can feel risky to be there—not in terms of your sobriety being at risk, but in terms of your actual physical safety being compromised. I do not choose to be in an enclosed space where an intoxicated individual is swinging a six-foot bullwhip, or a drunk bottom is flailing around the dungeon wearing stainless-steel manacles. Be who you are! Be proud to be sober, and don't compromise your sobriety or integrity for anyone. Ever."

Crazy Trans Woman Syndrome
Morgan M. Page

My doctor, who is a trans woman, and I had a conversation today about the guy who raped me earlier this year. At first she was like "did you charge him?" When I explained that he's a trans man of color, she immediately got why I hadn't. Not because I couldn't bear to put a trans person, especially a trans person of color, in jail (which I can't), but because it would cause me to be completely ostracized by the queer/trans community in Toronto. I'd be "just another crazy trans woman." It was an uncomfortable realization for both of us to sit there, as trans women, knowing that we have literally no recourse when violence is enacted on us within the community (though if the same violence conveniently came from a white cis straight man, we would be celebrated as heroes for standing up to such an easy target, at least within the queer/trans community).

She and I both, as professionals in the community, are well

aware of the fine line we have to walk in order to be taken seriously in the queer/trans community. We not only have to look a certain way (both in terms of passing and in terms of conforming to queer normative acceptable standards of appearance), we also have to make sure not to rock the boat too much. We have to appear as sane and calm as possible, no matter the circumstances. If we show too much emotion at any time (read: any inconvenient emotion), we get hit with a double whammy of misogyny and transphobia, quickly written off as hysterical "crazy trans women." Accuse the wrong person of something, anyone too close to queer-home, and that's the end of our credibility and the revoking of our entrance passes to Queerlandia.

It's exhausting having to walk such a fine line. I've found that there are so many "danger zones" to watch out for. Trans women have to not only be queer-literate (knowing queer social justice language), we have to be exceptionally good at using it. Any minor slip of language or politics and we're labeled "crazy trans women" by cis people while trans men nod knowingly in agreement—rarely standing up for us, and just as often perpetuating the "crazy trans woman" stereotype themselves.

I became aware of this initially through cryptic warnings from an older queer trans woman friend of mine, years before I became involved in the queer community, but I didn't realize the extent of it at first. That is, until I was invited to participate in it. When I first became involved heavily, I befriended two trans men whom I looked up to a great deal, and one of the first conversations we had in private was a gossip session in which they "warned" me about various trans women and got me to agree that they were "crazy." I've found similar conversations throughout the community, often used in a way that makes me wonder if what's really happening is that they're subconsciously testing my loyalty to the queer zeitgeist. Am I a good tranny or a bad tranny? Am I willing to be part of their clique, giving them the ability to deflect any and all criticism of transmisogyny, or am I a "problem"?

Before I realized that this was a system, that trans women were being systematically tested and written off, I engaged in it myself. You get a self-esteem boost, knowing that the cool kids don't count you among those trans women. Those trans women who stepped on the wrong toes, who take up "too much space," who don't have the right guilt-producing identity complex to be worthy of space (disabled young trans sex workers of color who vogue are considered highly prized friend-accessories, to be seen but not really heard beyond the occasional "gurl" for comedic effect, but only if they have the right haircut and the right clothes and are working towards a bachelors of gender studies or similarly useless degree).

Who are these "crazy trans women"? Often they are incredibly sincere activists who haven't had the privilege of being taught all of the ins and outs of anti-oppression social justice practice that is a prerequisite to membership in this queer community. Often they are labeled "too emotional" and "too angry," "loose cannons" who are out of control when speaking about our experiences of sex work that don't fit into the easily digestible "I do queer feminist porn on weekends to pay for my Fluevogs while I'm in grad school" vision of sex work that the queer community has deemed acceptable. Often they are trans women who are said to take up "too much space," while everyone whispers about how "you know, I know it's wrong to say, but she just seems like she has male privilege, you know? Like you can just feel it. Not that I'm saying she's a man, but, you know, you never know."

At the end of the day, this whole complex of issues is simply misogyny, ableism, and transphobia dressed up as "community accountability." It holds trans women to impossible standards, opening us up to vulnerability to all forms of in-community violence (physical, sexual, social), and creating a fear within the minds of so many queer trans women that our second-class position within the queer community could be ripped from our hands at any time for any minor infraction.

I'm tired of trying not to be a crazy trans woman in the voyeuristic eyes of the queer community.

Let's Talk About Interracial Porn
Jarrett Neal

Historical and cultural tensions surrounding issues of masculinity, race, violence, sexuality and miscegenation commix in both all-black and interracial pornography. Black men in gay porn customarily inhabit a position of power that has roots in racialized fetishism. To be blunt, black gay porn stars, when they are engaged in sex with white, Latino or Asian costars, almost always perform as "tops," the penetrative partner. Anatomically, these men possess athletic physiques, very dark skin, and penises that are much longer than the average five to seven inches most men's penises measure when erect. Dwight McBride states:

> In the all-black genre and in the blatino genre, black men are represented as "trade": men with hard bodies and hard personalities to match them, men from or tied to ghetto or street life in one way or another, men pos-

sessing exceptionally large penises...and, more often than not, men as sexual predators or aggressors.

Bobby Blake was a veteran black performer who, over the years, unleashed unbridled ultramasculine dominance over the many white men he had sex with on camera. A towering man with a solid Herculean physique, inky dark skin, plump lips and a broad nose, Blake has never been anally penetrated on camera. Blake maintained a long, successful career in gay porn and cultivated an avid fan base, but in 2000 he retired from the industry to become a minister. His stern, menacing appearance contrasts with those of black men who work in straight porn who must "be nonthreatening enough to appeal to...white men who [want] to jerk off to images of little virginal white girls being deflowered" (Poulson-Bryant). The black men hired to work in gay porn appear to be chosen for the opposite reason: the more threatening they appear and the larger their penises, the more popularity they garner.

Bobby Blake was no exception. His final film, *Niggas' Revenge,* boldly transgresses virtually every social, political and sexual taboo in Western culture. Blake, along with two other African-American co-stars, exacts revenge on a small group of backwoods white racists by imprisoning, torturing and sodomizing them. The actors in this film inhabit their roles convincingly, shouting racial epithets and embodying the worst stereotypes of both African-American and Caucasian men. The marriage of extreme cruelty and outré sex in *Niggas' Revenge,* which includes BDSM, fisting, urolangia and biastophilia, rather than making me feel uncomfortable, tantalized me. Sex aside, language is much more provocative than most sex acts and has the potential to cause more damage to an individual. Not only does *Niggas' Revenge* confirm the deep-seated beliefs of closet racists, it "referenc[es] the ugly historical and ideological realities out of which [black and gay sexual identities] have been formed" (Reid-Pharr). The verbal assault in *Niggas' Revenge*—even the title, which supposes a white racist gaze—is far more incendiary and repugnant than the debauchery that takes place on screen. Unlike the all-black genre of gay pornography, interracial gay pornography has the potential to provoke hostile encounters among its participants simply because it stubbornly relies on a white patriarchal rendering of black male sexuality and the full inventory of racist stereotypes ascribed to black men to fuel the lust of participants and viewers alike.

The catalogue of black gay porn, in which all of the participants are of African descent, ascribes to conventions that are common in gay porn: straight male seduction, muscle worship, and exhibitionism can all be found in gay porn specifically marketed to a black viewership. Yet leather, bear, and fetish porn for black men is nonexistent: these films make no distinction between races. Any black men who perform in these films do so alongside men of other races and ethnicities. Moreover, black gay porn includes scenarios that are not found in porn for Caucasian, Latino or Asian gays. In all-black films issues of class—the street thug conquering the middle-class black male, for example—and economic and social stratifications abound. The thug, outfitted in baggy jeans, an oversized white T-shirt and Timberland boots, has become the twenty-first century's symbol of reckless and raw masculine sexual energy. As such, he appeals to many gay men regardless of their race, economic or social status. He is viewed as rebellion incarnate, a repository of the culture's racial tensions and sexual repression.

Some young black gay men, motivated by a desire to distance themselves from the rampant homophobia that exists within the African-American community, have adopted the homo-thug façade as a means of declaring their masculinity while simultaneously embracing their desire for same-sex sex. Yet these men are loath to classify themselves as gay or bisexual. As a result, some engage in "down low" behavior. According to Keith Boykin, "the hypermasculinity of hip hop culture...created the homo-thug and the down low." The glorification of criminality, misogyny and homophobia endorsed by hip-hop artists through not only their lyrics but their lifestyle as well serves as the standard by which a sizable population of young black men gauges their masculinity. The homo-thug embodies qualities that make him a social and sexual outlaw. He has the ability to cross sexual boundaries and maintain his masculinity by dint of his racial classification and his ability to perform an unimpeachable version of masculinity, possessing "a fantastic insatiable animal sexuality that will fuck you tirelessly and still be ready for more" (McBride).

The homo-thug presents white-collar gay white men with an opportunity to indulge their lust without leaving the insular world they inhabit. By viewing interracial gay porn, gay white men who purposely distance themselves from genuine relationships with African-American men can indulge their private sexual fantasies while allowing racist and stereotypical beliefs regarding black men to persist. As bell hooks observes, "Euro-Americans seeking to leave behind a history of their brutal torture, rape, and enslavement of black bodies [project] all their fears onto black bodies." Even middle- and upper-class African-American gay men long to be sexually dominated by the homo-thug, who functions as a catalyst for their reclamation of an essential notion of blackness that they have tossed aside. The fetishization of the black male body, hence the black penis, emblemizes hypersexuality and masculine dominance while reinforcing the racist notion of white supremacy.

Gay pornography is considered a specialty market in the adult entertainment industry. Naturally, it appeals to a much smaller segment of the population, yet within this subdivision of the industry exists a multitude of studios that provide a sexual outlet for the desires of gay and bisexual men. The major studios film in scenic locations and employ only the most handsome and physically fit models. Each studio caters to the specific tastes of gay and bisexual men on the basis of fetish (e.g., leather, BDSM, barebacking) or a particular type of model. Falcon Studios primarily showcases white men, either boyish and ectomorphic or athletic and in their prime, between the ages of eighteen and thirty-five. Colt Studios specializes in films starring steroid-pumped bodybuilders over the age of thirty. Titan Media, perhaps the most sophisticated of the studios, regularly casts burly men over thirty. The cadre of men under contract with Titan Media crosses racial, ethnic and international lines, though Caucasian men make up the largest section of Titan models. The cast of men who perform in Titan Media films range from beefy, hairy DILFs to heavily tattooed counterculture punks to preppie clean-shaven men who represent what is commonly called the "all-American" look. Since 1995, Titan Media has been highly successful in luring viewers into a fantasy world populated by rugged, stunningly handsome men with overdeveloped physiques who fuck each other wildly in implausible scenarios.

At the beginning of the millennium, Titan Media introduced a new star to its films. His demeanor and his frankly aggressive sexual performance set him apart from other Titan Media stars and other black performers in general. Dred Scott is unlike any other man in gay porn. Of indeterminate origins—virtually no information can be obtained regarding his private life—Dred Scott's looks and temperament inspire as much fear as they do lust. Scott first appeared in the Titan Media film *Fallen Angel IV: Sea Men* in 2003. The star of the film, inspired by Jean Genet's seminal gay novel *Querelle of Brest*, Scott plays a seaman roaming a docked freighter dressed only in dark pants, suspenders, work boots and a black beanie as he engages in a variety of sex acts with fellow seamen. Part of Titan's fetish collection, *Fallen Angel IV: Sea Man* showcases Scott as he exhibits his penchant for aggressive sex, violent thrusting, slapping and rough language, elements that would later become Dred Scott's trademark. In the Titan Media feature *Trespass,* Scott plays an escaped convict on the lam from several groups of bounty hunters (all of them white) who seek to recapture him. He scrambles through the wilderness shackled and handcuffed, dressed in a blue prisoner's uniform in search of new clothes and a tool to cut his bonds. Once he finds bolt cutters and new clothes, free at last, he has his way with a brawny bounty hunter (Patrick Knight) in the bed of the latter's pickup truck. *Slammer,* a film that takes place in prison, opens with Scott, acting as the prison warden, subjecting a wiry new inmate, Billy Wild, to violent sex and verbal abuse while a guard watches, aroused.

No single aspect of Dred Scott's persona can sufficiently capture what distinguishes him from his African-American peers. Perhaps the one thing that makes him different is that he has never been marketed as a black performer. Titan Media's other major black performers of the 2000s, Ben Jakks and Diesel Washington, had no choice but to be marketed in a way that confined them to essential and often stereotypical characterizations of black masculinity, and both appeared only in interracial films. In almost all of their films they were the only black males who star in the film, and they never shared sex scenes with other black performers. Ben Jakks, who is British, has unblemished bronze skin, no tattoos, a bald head and a basketball player's sleek physique. In his five Titan films, he was often cast as a mysterious seducer. His sex scenes are imbued with a sensuousness that most pornographic films lack, and his approach to his costars—typically boyish white men—is tender and nonthreatening. Diesel Washington, for a time the reigning black performer for Titan, is an avatar of the ferocious black stud realized by Bobby Blake. His name—a combination of the surnames of actors Vin Diesel and Denzel Washington—trumpets his embrace of these two performers, one an action-film star of multiracial extraction and the other a critically acclaimed black actor working in mainstream cinema. Diesel Washington made ten movies for Titan since he began working for the studio in the mid-2000s. In his films he performs as a strict top. Like Ben Jakks, Diesel Washington is tall and lithe, yet in contrast to Jakks's seductive image, Washington's persona, buttressed by his heavily tattooed dark skin and sexual prowess, bears more relation to the homo-thug. While Jakks presents a version of black masculinity that is genteel and rather cosmopolitan, Washington fully embraces the stereotype of the menacing, hostile black man located squarely in the ghetto fantasies of Titan's largely gay white audience.

Completing the trio of top black performers exclusively contracted with Titan Media during this period is the enigmatic Dred Scott. Though not seductive like Ben Jakks or as easily categorized as a homo-thug like Diesel Washington, Dred Scott, given his obvious multiracial background—the word *Black* is tattooed on his right pectoral, and the word *White* is tattooed on his left, both in Old English type—was allowed more access into the erotic fantasy world of Titan Media. Dred Scott's stage name evokes the United States' original sin of slavery, mixing his viewers' erotic imagination with the destructive legacy of racism. However we may object to this rationale or protest against it "race is a salient variable in the sex-object choices we make in the gay marketplace of desire...[and] those who benefit unduly under such a system (whites) have a great deal invested in depoliticizing desire" (McBride). Given his racial blend, the fury contained in his facial expressions, his manic thrusting during sexual intercourse and his penchant for sadomasochism, one can easily imagine Scott as a vengeful mulatto conceived during the rape of a slave woman by her white master.

The real Dred Scott was born a slave in Virginia approximately two decades after the founding of the United States. He is famous for having unsuccessfully sued his master for his freedom, in a Supreme Court case now known as the *Dred Scott Decision*, which held that his bondage to his master remained in force even in territories where slavery was illegal. Under the weight of such massive historical, racial, cultural and sexual systems, it is impossible not to draw a number of conclusions regarding gay porn star Dred Scott's function within the sphere of erotic entertainment, and the messages, whether intentional or not, that he wishes viewers to glean from his work. Notwithstanding the various motives that might come into play, including financial ones—it has been suggested that Dred Scott was a heterosexual man who did gay porn because it paid better than straight—it seems unlikely that he would adopt the name of one of the nation's most heroic African-American men without being aware of its implications. If our sexual desires are in essence a manifestation of our hidden needs and fears, they can also subsume our hatred and disgust. By reincarnating Dred Scott the slave, Dred Scott the porn star was communicating to viewers that our erotic ideation cannot be divorced from historical, political and cultural realities.

"Because of the legacy of white supremacy and its persistence in the form of white American racism, the notions we have evolved of what stands as beautiful and desirable are thoroughly racialized," wrote Dwight A. McBride (2005). "[O]ur ideas about aesthetics in the broadest sense are shot through with racial considerations that render attempts at depoliticizing them impossible." Unlike his forebear Bobby Blake or his colleagues Ben Jakks and Diesel Washington, Dred Scott's appearance—skin the color of butter pecan ice cream, an aquiline nose, rippling muscles, a stubble-shaved head, reddish-brown facial hair and a torso clad in black tattoos that resemble armor—is more closely aligned with notions of white male beauty. This affords him the opportunity to traverse realms of sexual exchange in areas of gay erotica into which few men of color are allowed to venture. In essence, Scott's light skin serves as currency even more than his penis or ferocious sexual energy. Although Scott's African-American ancestry is unquestionable, it is equally clear that he has Caucasian genes. Similar to house slaves in the antebellum South, Scott is white enough for his white costars, producers and directors to grant him entry into a rarefied space among the elite of gay porn, yet still black enough to keep him at a distance from his fans, white and black alike, as an archetype of the homo-thug.

Despite this license to enhance his homo-thug image, Dred Scott is still bound to the narrowly defined roles assigned to black men in gay porn. He performs on camera as an exclusive top, often exhibiting a domineering, hypermasculine persona. In the seven Titan Media films he starred in, he subjected his submissive white and Latino partners to verbal abuse, slapping, spitting, body slamming and urination. These acts are not uncommon in mainstream gay porn: sexual acts that were once confined to specialty or fetish films have gradually encroached into more popular productions. At some point in their careers, porn actors of all races and ethnicities participate in aberrant forms of sexual expression on camera. Bobby Blake in *Niggas' Revenge* displayed behaviors far more sadistic than any that Dred Scott engaged in on camera, yet his character in *Niggas' Revenge* operates within a system of sexual debauchery alive with racist and homophobic extremism. The entire film glories in depravity.

The sadomasochism that Dred Scott enacts upon his costars appears to come from an ambiguous place of rage, once again owing to his resistance to racial and ethnic classification. When Bobby Blake abuses white men in *Niggas' Revenge*, viewers know without a doubt that the "rage" he expresses, as the title promises, is racial at root. Dred Scott is often cast as an anonymous drifter in his films. He speaks very little dialogue and, in keeping with the element of fantasy in these films, he embarks on sexual odysseys in which he alone determines the narrative course of action and which sex acts will be performed. Yet his sexual prowess and dominance do not obviate his limited function within gay porn. Despite Dred Scott's ability to alter and expand the homo-thug archetype, he is still bound to its strictures: he is never the object of seduction in these scenarios, and he is never sexually passive with white men.

The sexual dominance exercised over white men speaks volumes about Dred Scott's body as a site where historical, racial and masculine systems converge. And yet, like all African-American men engaged in gay pornography, he is confined to a role that forces black men to avoid expressing any authentic homosexual desire. McBride continues: "The ideological lessons taught and propagated by [such] films are that white men have sex with black men for reasons having to do with master fantasies and power, retributive sex…or to trade on their value as currency in the gay marketplace of desire." Black men bottoming for white men on camera remains a taboo in films produced by major gay adult studios such as Titan.

Western culture's insistence on preserving the Mandingo myth, and its propagation in films, television programs, advertisements and homophobic hip-hop lyrics, makes it difficult for men in the gay marketplace of desire to feel comfortable with the idea of black men, especially hypermasculine black men like Dred Scott, sexually submitting to white men. To some extent this discomfort stems from the belief that white men topping black men is somehow inherently racist, an idea that harks back to the same tensions surrounding pornographic scenarios involving white men and black women. But this argument has more to do with power than race. In his incendiary, vituperative and fiercely homophobic rants in *Soul on Ice*, Eldridge Cleaver lambastes black gay homosexuals, claiming that we have a racial death wish as expressed in the act of being sexually submissive with white men. Since white men, by and large, hold political and economic power in Western culture, in the realm of erotic desire a reversal of roles, where black men hold dominance and white men must submit to them, balances the power differential. Yet as African-American men gain political and economic power (as evidenced chiefly by the election of Barack Obama as the nation's first black president) the dynamics that have traditionally ordered gay erotica and pornography are slowly evolving.

While the major studios continue to resist sexually subordinating black men to white men, smaller and emerging studios are producing some interracial gay porn in which black men bottom for white men. Planta Rosa Productions, which specializes in gonzo bareback films (unscripted films that involve unprotected anal sex), features black men—primarily Brazilian and Afro-Caribbean—who perpetuate the Mandingo stereotype, but it balances these scenes with others in which black men are topped by white ones. In all of these scenarios, the white top is a performer who goes by the mononym Igor. Well-endowed, lanky and hairy, with dark circles beneath his eyes, Igor mugs for the camera whenever he performs, contorting his face in a variety of goofy expressions as he thrusts and ruts inside of his costars, black and white alike, with gleeful abandon. White porn star and director Marco Paris performs almost exclusively with black men, though he assumes both active and passive roles. What is interesting about this inversion of the norm is that the tops in these cases are not American: Igor is Russian and Marco Paris is Slovakian. The fact that only European white men are allowed to sexually dominate men of African descent highlights the insidiousness of racism that pervades American society and the comfort black men feel sexually submitting to white men who are not descended from slave-owning ancestors.

The black male body historically has served both as a repository of Western culture's most ardent and prurient desires, and its hatred and disgust of racial and sexual "others." Dred Scott's career in gay pornography ended as quickly and mysteriously as it began. After making seven films with Titan Media, he had no further public engagement with erotic entertainment. Dred Scott may have freed himself from the need to do gay porn, but his persona on camera remains captive to the social systems that perpetuate racist and homophobic myths and stereotypes regarding African-American men and gay men. The paradox of acquiring fame within the gay adult entertainment industry is no more or less problematic for Dred Scott than it is for all men of color. In an era when those who inhabit the ultraconservative fringe continue to lob racist attacks at President Obama, the de facto symbol of black masculinity in the twenty-first century, even as the gay rights movement is gaining greater support among Americans, I find it damning that our culture is still unwilling to relinquish its addiction to destructive, shameful and anachronistic representations of black gay sexuality. Perhaps Dred Scott felt the same way and refused to contribute to it any longer. Of course the answer may never be known. And as the social and sexual paradigms that once ordered gay pornography rapidly change, as the major studios alter their films to keep pace not only with web-based production companies such as Tim Tales and Men at Play but also swift cultural changes within the gay community, redefinitions and realignments of all sorts will be necessary.

References:

Boykin, Keith. *Beyond the Down Low: Sex, Lies, and Denial in Black America*. Carroll & Graff, 2005.

Cleaver, Eldridge. *Soul on Ice*. Ramparts, 1968.

hooks, bell. *We Real Cool: Black Men and Masculinity*. Routledge, 2004.

McBride, Dwight A. *Why I Hate Abercrombie & Fitch: Essays on Race and Sexuality*. NYU Press, 2005.

Poulson-Bryant, Scott. *Hung: A Meditation on the Measure of Black Men in America*. Doubleday, 2005 .

Reid-Pharr, Robert F. *Black Gay Man: Essays*. NYU Press, 2001.

When I Was a Birthday Present for an Eighty-Two-Year-Old Grandmother
David Henry Sterry

"David, I've got a fantastic job for you, Friday night, this is a two-hundred-dollar job!" Mr. Hartley's straight-shooter baritone reaches down my throat all the way to my seventeen-year-old balls and squeezes hard.

"Wow," I say in what I hope is a loverstudguy voice, but which I suspect smacks of eunuch, "that's great, excellent, thanks, I uh—"

"David," Mr. Hartley sounds like a benevolent dictator in a three-piece suit, the ultimate Master Alpha, "this is a very important client. And if you do this job well I can absolutely guarantee there will be lots of exciting opportunities on the horizon for you. You understand me, David? Do we understand each other?"

I have no idea what he's talking about so I say:

"Sure, absolutely, I got it—"

"This is a very unique opportunity for you, David. I want you to be completely prepared. It's a rather unusual job. But I think it really matches your skill set."

My brain races like a train on bad speed. Will there be barnyard animals involved? Ritual sacrifice? Death masks and scat sandwiches? What will you do for money? Where do you draw your line? How much of your life are you willing to sell for two hundred dollars?

"David, this client, who I must emphasize is extremely important, has decided she wants to treat her friend to a very special birthday gift. And that birthday gift is you. So get ready to put on your birthday suit." Mr. Hartley laughs like a machine gun: rat-a-tat-tat. "I kid of course. Seriously though, David, it's our policy at the Hollywood Employment Agency to give our clients all the information they need to succeed. We believe that preparation is essential to success. And for this job, it's very important that you understand you are being given by one of our most important clients to her best friend, as a present for her eighty-second birthday."

GULP!

"It's very important to us that our clients are comfortable performing. Are you comfortable, under the circumstances, uh... performing...David?"

No. No. No. I don't honestly think I can fuck an eighty-two-year-old. That's what I say in my seventeen-year-old man-child idiot head. Out loud I say:

"Sure, absolutely, I'm all over it."

"You're all over it." Mr. Hartley's Uzi of a laugh rattles my skull. "That is droll, David, very droll. That's exactly why I thought of you when this job came in. I have every confidence that you won't let me...down." Bam bam bam, Mr. Hartley laughs fast and staccato. "I kid of course. David, I want you to call me as soon as this job is done. Do you understand? Do we understand each other?"

"Absolutely, for sure, yeah."

Mr. Hartley gives me the 411 and then I disconnect.

Immediately my shattered brain sees an ancient naked wrinkled saggy droopy granny spread-eagled in front of me and my poor placid flaccid penis is a lifeless piece of useless meat, I have to give the money back; I see myself spiraling down humiliated, a brutal failure rejected by Mr. Hartley and Sunny, drummed out of the business shunned by all my chicken peers the only family I know at this point who accepts me for what I am, my paycheck my refuge my people, all gone.

Anonymously knocking on the door in the ultra-fancy ass swank swish hotel that smells like Olde Money, my mind attacks itself with vicious visions of wrinkled, ravaged, sagging grandmother flesh that shrink-wrap my rapidly shriveling penis. Breath short. Tight. Heart racehorsing pounding against my breastplate. A sticky clammy sweaty nervy jumpy freaky tweaky moisture oozes out of most of my pores.

The door slowly opens. She's trim and pretty in pink and a styly Chanel-type suit. She definitely has one of those helmet hairdos, but it's well done if you like that kind of thing. A huge honking diamond ring holds court on a well-tended finger. Shoes the same color pink as her outfit. She's got wrinkles but they're not gruesome. She's wearing makeup but it's definitely not Whatever-Happened-to-Baby-Janey. But the best thing about her is her smile. She has a smile that welcomes you in. After a heavy sigh full of deep relief the first thought that pops into my seventeen-year-old man-child head is: *Shit man, I hope I'm doing this good when I'm eighty-two years old.*

Like a hostess greeting an international dignitary, she asks me if I would like some champagne? Chocolate-covered strawberries? Pâté and cheese? It's all spread out on this fancy silvery tray.

Curtains are closed. Lights are low. Candlelight makes everything soft. She gives me a long thin beautiful flute of champagne. With a sweet smile ripe with kindness. Like I'm all growed up. I know what to do. I've been trained well by my mum.

"I want to wish you a very, very happy birthday, and if there's anything I can do to make your dreams come true, I'm here for your pleasure."

I have rehearsed the speech. I am pleased with the delivery. I hold up the long thin beautiful flute of sparkly bubbly. She smiles kinda shy. Demure. Which is shockingly endearing in a lady who's turning out to be the totally awesome grandma I never had. That I'm just about to have sex with.

She holds out her flute for a clink. Weak clink. We drink. The champagne shoots little giddy meteors tickling my lips and teasing my nose. I love the way it feels inside my mouth like the most sophisticated pop rocks ever. Smooth smooth, smooth, it goes down tingly and frothy, liquid laughter.

She tells me her name is Dorothy. But her friends called her Dot. I think that's a cool name. Dot. She's talking about the champagne. Apparently she knows a lot about champagne. This is from some famous champagne place in France. Soon as I'm done with the first sip I can't wait for another so I just let it guzzle down my muzzle all twinkly and sparkly. One more big gulp and the whole beautiful flute is empty, the contents now inside me. It comes on quick and suddenly my head floats on my neck and my face is happy, bones melting, blood rushing like carefree debutantes jitterbugging at their coming-out ball. It feels a lot greater to be alive than it did five minutes ago.

Dot insists I have a chocolate-covered strawberry. Doesn't take much arm-twisting. Apparently it's some world-famous chocolate from Belgium. It's got a hard crunch when you bite it, but then it gets all melty in your mouth, as the fruity juice of the rapturously ripe strawberry sings with the chocolate in mind-boggling two-part harmony. When I finish I see Dot watching me with a big grin on her face. Makes me like her. Even more. Dot tells me she likes to watch people enjoy themselves. I tell her how much I'm enjoying myself. And the crazy thing is I completely mean it. She asks me if I want another one. I say no, even though I really actually do want another one. She asks me if I really want another one but I'm just saying no to be polite. Like she can see right inside my head. I confess I do and did. She insists with an impish grin that I have another chocolate-covered strawberry. So I do. I have two more after that. I could eat every single one. But I am there to do a job. I figure after three chocolate-covered strawberries, it might impair my ability to perform.

Dot tells me all about her madcap romantic husband, how they met, how he proposed to her. Took her to Europe, South America, Broadway shows. She hauls out a picture of him. It's black-and-white. He's in a sharp suit with two-tone shoes, hair all slick and a debonair devilmaycare smile. I must admit, he was one dapper motherfucker.

He's been dead for ten years. It's sad and happy at the same time. Makes me like her so much that she has all this love for this guy she was married to for like fifty years or whatever. Being now the son of a dyke from a home broken beyond repair and having sex for money with grandmothers, I just can't fathom being married to somebody for fifty years. But Dot says her old man was a pistol and a mensch and a big old bundle of fun. Dot tells me about how they used to have these wild and crazy parties with all their brilliant zany friends, where they'd get all dressed up, drinking, dancing and yakking all night about art and politics and life and death and war and taxes.

It's a mad blast listening to her wax about her one wild and precious life. Makes me hope that at some point I can have one. A life. A most excellent wife, some brilliant crazy zany friends, a house with a pool and lots of rooms where people can party. Sounds nice.

This is such a great job so far. But of course there's that nagging tug in the back and pit of my head and belly: how in the name of Pan the horny goat boy am I going to get It up and off? I am bombarded by the image of my meat torpedo morphing into wet spaghetti. I am forced to focus extra hard to avoid hyperventilation.

Dot stops talking. She hems and she haws and she tuts. Clearly she wants to tell me what's on the menu for her birthday dinner, but she's having a terrible time spitting it out.

I'm scared breathless. I desperately want to give Dot what she wants. I need to please her. She's been so nice to me. And I want to succeed at this job. Be an American. Be a man. But will I be able to achieve liftoff with a naked octogenarian lying on top of me? I believe I can. I know I can't. What if she wants to do some weird old person sex thing I don't know about?

My testes cower in a corner. My head is like a balloon being inflated by a homicidal clown with ADHD. My guts rumble thunderously, roiling like a boiler about to blow.

Again I find myself seriously questioning my career choice.

Dot forces out a strangulated sentence like a tongue-tied eighty-two-year-old schoolgirl.

"I've always wanted someone to kiss me..." she motions with her head down towards her nether regions, "down there."

That's it? Thank you Lord, for delivering me from the wilderness. A little head? A wee dram of cunnilingus? Hell, I can do that with my eyes closed. In fact many times I have. And then I think, *Can you imagine wanting to have someone go down on you for fifty years? Having a husband you love and not being able to ask him to do that?* I've gone down on every girlfriend I've ever had. It seems like one of the most basic sexual things you can do. My mind is officially boggled.

But the weight of the world, so heavy on my head moments ago, has been mercifully lifted. I assure Dot that I would be more than happy to make her dream come true.

She gets under the covers. She doesn't take her clothes off. This is just getting better and better.

Here are the best jobs in order:

1) Just talking.
2) Just talking while I'm naked.
3) Just talking while I'm naked and playing with myself. And by playing with myself of course I mean masturbating.
4) Cunnilingussing.
5) Doggy styling.
6) Missionary positioning.
7) Cowgirling with direct eye contact.

So this is the fourth best job there is.

Dot wiggles and wriggles under the covers. I assume she's taking her granny panties off. She doesn't tell me to take my clothes off so I don't. I crawl under the covers. I suspect there will be wrinkly grandmother flesh. But what do I care? Cunnilingus is cunnilingus. Luckily I was trained in this art by the first girl-friend I ever had, who was much older than me and rigorously demanding, albeit in a very sweet educational way.

So it takes a while for me to burrow myself in, but eventually there I am. Right between Dot's eighty-two-year-old legs. It's very dark in there. Like a cave. I like it. And when I arrive, to my surprise it smells good. Fresh. Manicured. Everything is quite smooth leading up to the area. Which is a very pleasant surprise. Dot is very ironing-board-like. But cunnilingually I've been trained well. I take my time. I go slow. I kiss all around the area soft and gentle. Some lips. A little tongue. Very light. The more I do it the more she softens. Then suddenly she's moving herself towards my mouth. Now there are little moans and sighs and groans and gasps coming from outside the covers. How cool is this? I'm thinking, she's totally into it.

At this moment I feel so useful.

Her hands are on my head and she's pulling it into her area. And to tell you the truth, her area is much like any other area I've been in. Especially in the depth of this black cave.

Dot is now gently manipulating my head, moving it exactly where she wants it and I'm just applying the appropriate pressure. It's like we're dancing and she's leading while I follow. And she's exhibiting all the symptoms of excitation. It's all happening and I could not be happier.

Dot now seems to be climbing the ladder of the stairway to Heaven. I don't know how long we been going at this now, but it doesn't seem that long. And she's already manifesting all the physical manifestations of pre-orgasm.

Sure enough, here it comes. Here she comes.

Here comes Dot. Diving off the cliff into the sea of sexual ecstasy.

I am overpowered by a sense of joyful satisfaction. Mr. Hartley will be so proud of me.

It's clear we are, you know, done. So I burrow out from undercover and head into the bathroom, to give her a chance to put herself back together. As I eyeball myself in the mirror, I shake my seventeen-year-old man-child idiot head. Can you imagine? Eighty-two-year-old grandmother pussy tasted great.

Sure enough, when I come back out, she's totally put together, like nothing happened. Except for the bloom in her cheeks and the sweet smile of satisfaction on her lips. Dot thanks me profusely. She asks me if I would like to take a chocolate-covered strawberry with me. I confess that I would. I grab a chocolate-covered strawberry and head for the door full to overflowing with a sense of well-being. Even though my parents don't care to speak to me, even though I have no home and no family except for a bunch of prostitutes and a pimp, even though I have no future and I'm wracked by nightmares and lusting for revenge on the man who attacked and broke me into tattered pieces, at least I'm good at this.

As I'm leaving with my chocolate-covered strawberry Dot surreptitiously slips a crisp green bill into my hand while she plants a very nice kiss on my cheek. When I pull back, she playfully wipes the lipstick off my cheek. It's a tiny little gesture, but it feels so intimate and connected in a world where connection is virtually impossible for me.

I thank her profusely—wish her a happy birthday.

She thanks me right back.

Then I'm gone.

It's a hundred dollar bill. Add that to the two hundred that was in the envelope on the fancy food platter. So that's three hundred dollars to drink fancy French champagne, eat world-famous Belgian chocolate-covered strawberries and make one pretty great grandma's dream come true.

As I leave the ultra-swank Beverly Hills Hotel, I find myself thinking:

America, what a country!

What an Armpit Model Taught Me about Sexual Language
Jon Pressick

"I love it when the guy fucks me in my armpit, cum[s] there, etc. My per-
sonal dream is to realize a movie with nine men in one interesting Tantric
position in which one of them fucks my pussy, another one my ass and a
third in my mouth. One more is between the feet, two more in the armpits,
one between the boobs and two hand jobs for two others. I think it would
be very beautiful and magic."

My jaw fell open, my heart raced and I had a minor panic
attack. I looked through the glass and saw my producer's face
reflect mine. And my next guest, a well-known sex writer, had
her hands on her cheeks, eyes wide and mouth extended in an
"Ohhhhhhh!" I could see but not hear.

And it went on. And on. I was live on community radio with
a guest describing, in great detail, how and what she would do
with nine men at one time.

I had been one of the hosts of "Sex City" on the University of Toronto's radio station CIUT 89.5FM for about three years. While it is community radio, and firmly entrenched there, CIUT actually transmits a far-reaching signal that travels a 150km radius around the city. It definitely isn't something you have to hold an antenna out the window on a clear day to receive. CIUT is a well-known, well-respected station and "Sex City" has been a part of the station for more than fifteen years.

While the station itself is run by volunteers and managed by a few paid staff, it ultimately has to answer to the same government body as all other Canadian broadcasters: the Canadian Radio Telecommunications Commission (CRTC). That agency has many functions, including ensuring compliance to Canadian Content requirements, granting broadcasting licenses and ensuring community broadcast standards.

But this is Canada. We really don't hear of many incidents where broadcasters are admonished for breaching community broadcast standards. Once in a while a shockjock will come along, say something offensive and be fined. But that is rare. Most of our content is as quaint as you'd expect.

Over the years, "Sex City" has actually received one notice of complaint. The mandate of the show is to discuss sex, sexuality and gender as they relate to current affairs, social issues, politics, the arts and much more. "Sex City" explores a simple theme that has a wide base of content from which to draw. While it varies between our four to five hosts, the general setup of the show is to interview a few guests and in between segments, we play a few sexy songs that fit the theme of the show.

But it wasn't anything we said; it was one of those songs that led to someone in the community calling in a complaint to the CRTC. Sure, we discuss fetish, sex worker rights, erotica…but it was "I Don't Give A…" by Peaches that was just too much for one listener. Because it was just one call, there was no formal admonishment or penalty, but from that point on, we knew that people were listening and that we might piss them off.

The "I Don't Give A…" incident happened a couple of years before I started on the show, but it did happen when we were still in our 5:00 p.m. Saturday afternoon time slot. It is not a coveted spot, with people mostly listening in their cars. Still, it was better than Wednesday afternoon, the show's original airtime.

At three years in, I was comfortable on the mic, I was booking strong and interesting guests and I was always conscious of the line we have to toe when it comes to the sensitive nature of sexual topics. I have a standard speech of what words can and cannot be said on air. We need guests to understand and hopefully heed this because CIUT does not have a delay and our producers cannot bleep offensive language. If we say it, you will hear it. No take backs.

Because I was feeling good, I was really branching out on subject matter and guests. Researching people and their widely ranging sexual interests and activities is fascinating stuff. I want to challenge myself and my listeners and bring topics into conversation that do not normally get spoken of.

That ethos gave me the really good idea of interviewing a Russian armpit fetish model.

I don't even remember how I came across Bestia or even the idea of armpit fetish. I've seen and heard of a lot of different porn, but maschalagnia (armpit fetishism) was entirely new to me. But once I found Bestia, found some of the sites and magazines she had appeared in and on, I thought it would make for a unique and intriguing discussion on the show.

I mentioned that she is Russian, right?

Connecting over email, she explained that her understanding of English is very strong—written English that is. She explained that she can speak English, but not well enough to carry a conversation, particularly with radio nerves getting in the way. So we concocted a plan wherein I provided her the interview questions so that she could prepare her responses in advance, practice reading them and then recite them back to me while we were live on the air.

This seemed a straightforward approach so I went ahead, produced the questions and sent them off to her. She was grateful for my consideration and promised to prepare great answers. She did, however, offer one caveat: she told me to not deviate from our "script." If I were to ad-lib or throw in a new question, she would potentially freeze up and lose her place in the interview. I appreciated her candor and readily agreed. We were all set.

Unfortunately, I made two mistakes.

Show day came and I was feeling good. I was excited, feeling that I was going to do something edgy and one-of-a-kind. I was really looking forward to talking with Bestia! Through my intrepid research, I'd developed an interest in her work and this always makes an interview better. Plus, I was on pins and needles waiting to hear what Bestia had prepared.

Mistake #1: I did not request to read her responses. I didn't even think of it. I am still not entirely convinced it was necessary, but listening to that interview again, I really should have. None of our guests are outrageous with their talk. Maybe it is because of the language speech. That talk is a pretty clear indicator that our conversation needs to be family friendly—even when dealing with sexual themes.

Mistake #2: I didn't give Bestia that language speech. In a lapse of thought and judgment I just assumed she wouldn't even know English sexual colloquialisms. Unlike not vetting her responses, this mistake was an actual choice I made.

So, a few questions in, she launched into that desired epic sex act and I was aghast. I didn't know what to do. As the words came out of her mouth in Ukraine and out over the air in Canada and beyond, I felt my fun, hobby radio career hitting a brick wall of censure. From the station. From the CRTC. From the rest of the "Sex City" crew for screwing up so badly.

I thought about stopping her. I thought about jumping to the next question. I wondered if she'd understand what I was doing and roll with it or if she really would be completely flummoxed. Earlier on in my "Sex City" career I had done some pretty bad interviews. Ones where I completely lost—or never had—the guest. In one instance, an overly nervous artist replied with nothing but one-word answers. That experience was horrible and I really didn't want to get into a situation where Bestia was confused.

So I let her continue, uninterrupted, in all her armpit orgy glory.

After the show we were all, understandably, taken aback. The common sentiment was that we hoped, this one time, that no one was listening. That, I tell you, is an odd feeling for a producer of media content. But I really was afraid that we would get in trouble. Can you imagine a parent, channel-hopping with a car full of kids, pressing the scan button and having it land on a station just as "one of them fucks my pussy, another one my ass and a third in my mouth" comes out of the speakers?

To be clear, never have I held any of this against Bestia. It all falls on me. I did not perform my due diligence about language and I did not review her material. She was very professional and did much to promote her appearance both before it aired and after. She often mentioned the interview online, well after it aired. Had I discussed the parameters with her, I have no doubt she'd have been amenable. We have had guests who flagrantly violate our language requirements, but I am sure Bestia wouldn't do that. Luckily, we did manage to fly under the radar on this one. No complaints. Not from the community, not from the government, not from the station. Wipe that brow and give a big whistle! I did not want to inflict punishment on the station or my colleagues for these mistakes. And I wanted to remain on the air! But from that point on, I was certainly more cautious about who I booked and how I instructed them about their obligations of language.

The thing is...I really hate doing that.

When my first daughter was born, I had a conversation with her mother and a friend of mine about using coarse language around children. Personally, I have no issue with it as long as that language, when used, is given context and consideration. In other words, I would tell my kids what I mean by the word *fuck* and I would advise them with whom and where it is appropriate to discuss such words. At home? Sure. With family? Fine. With extended family? Not a good idea. At school? Hell no.

However, my ex (and my friend, surprisingly), did not agree with this philosophy, so we went the more traditional route of not swearing and teaching them to not swear as well. The funny thing is, had we gone with my cussin'-friendly idea, I would have had a much more challenging transition to talking on the radio. Because I curse. A lot. Sailors ain't got nothing on me. But I only do it when the kids aren't around. Now that they are in their teens, I have loosened the linguistic lasso a bit, but I am still guarded when it comes to what I say around them.

And that liberation feels so nice. I heartily believe we should be using the words that are comfortable to us. Certainly, be aware of meaning, use words in the right context—even if that context is just an expletive born out of frustration or difficulty. Everybody needs the occasional "Oh shit!" moment. Sometimes a naughty word is the only appropriate one that will fit the situation. And when it comes to sex, that is more often the case than not.

Another part of my parenting strategy has been to never shy away from my kids' questions about sex and sexuality. If they ask, I tell them. If something interesting comes up in culture or current events, I discuss it with them. In doing so, I think I have helped them to have positive attitudes about sex, sexuality and gender. We frequently visit the zoo and one time we saw two giant tortoises mating. All of the other parents around were giving their kids explanations about the animals playing leapfrog or some such nonsense. One of mine turned to me and said, "They're mating, right?"

Now, given that we were in a public place, I wouldn't have approved of her saying, "They're fucking, right?" And because my little language experiment was not endorsed by the full parental council of our home, I really don't know if I'd have approved of that comment at home. But the idea, to me, remains: Why do we hold such stock in perceived "dirty" words—particularly when it comes to sex? Did our control over their language stunt their development and understanding of sex...on their own terms?

Sometime after the Bestia interview, a funny coincidence became an ongoing situation. At some point, one guest used the word *cock* live on air. And then the next week and then the next...until it seemed as if cock had become a required part of the show. The funny thing is, cock wasn't said every week, but it did get used frequently enough, over an extended period, that we stopped noticing. What is, arguably, the male C-word (though I acknowledge not as loaded) became so commonplace on our show as to be indistinguishable from the rest of the conversations. And nary a complaint has been registered.

So, why can't this happen with the rest of the so-called dirty words? Would liberating *fuck, shit, cunt,* and the rest of their ilk actually free our tongues as well as our relationships with sex and sex-related topics?

We saw this happen on "Sex City" with cock. Radio and television have embraced *ass,* rescuing it from the unspeakable list. In a disturbingly parallel situation, actual anatomically correct words for genitalia have also been freed with some, such as *penis* and *vagina* heard more frequently in media and casual conversation. Can other words, sexual or not, be far behind?

Don't get me wrong; I certainly believe there are some words that should not come into common use. However, I cannot think of any of a sexual context that should be censored. The key here is context and intention. Sure, *cocksucker, slut* and *pervert* are most frequently used as insults and are meant to demean and harm. But that is just one context—not the version I am trumpeting. All three of those can also be used with the deepest of affection. Of course, *slut* and *pervert* are commonplace words, but they aren't accepted as positive descriptors.

Will it ever be possible, in a film or on TV, for an actor to say about another actor "What a cocksucker!" and mean it positively?

My observations of "Sex City" and popular media make me think we've already got this down in real life. The parlance of our times suggests that *fucking, cock, dick, balls, pussy, cunt* and *tits* are far more commonly used among lovers and friends than *intercourse,* *penis, vulva, vagina, breasts* and the rest of the biological terms. Somehow, those who actually talk about sex are more comfortable using alternative wording than they are hearing them. So while the more salacious words may not be the proper terms, they are at least creating conversations about sex.

I've since lost touch with Bestia. Her website is under repair. I wonder if she is still keen on armpits and having hers ravished... I wonder if she still models or if she's moved on to something new.... I wonder if she ever made that glorious gang bang happen.

What I wonder most of all is if she'd tell me, in a personal conversation, all about that wild orgy she happily told my listeners about. Armpits remain a fairly out-there fetish. Was she brave enough to talk about her interests in such a raunchy way because it had to do with performance? Would she be so bold if we were just sharing beer, chatting?

Raise your hand if you think she would.

Growing Through the Yuck

Ashley Manta

It is easy to get sucked into the negative when you're living with herpes. I remember the day that I was diagnosed. I was at the health center at my university and I had the most horrific first herpes outbreak anyone could imagine. Two solid weeks of not being able to sit, lie down, use the bathroom, or shower without excruciating pain. Not to mention the accompanying nausea, fatigue, and general feelings of misery. The nurse gave me the diagnosis and I felt my heart hit the floor.

Who would want me now since I have herpes? With shaking hands I dialed my then boyfriend's cell phone number. "The rash I have? It's herpes," I said, cringing with every word. "I had a feeling that's what it was," he replied calmly. "Are you mad?" I asked. "No, sweetie," he said, "you're still the same person you were an hour ago. It's just herpes. It's not life-threatening."

I was shocked. I was expecting anger—even fury. I spread

herpes to him unknowingly because I didn't recognize the symptoms, and here he was reassuring me! Together we researched home remedies and information on herpes that was now a part of both of our lives. We supported each other through our first outbreak and subsequent herpes outbreaks, until we finally went our separate ways a few months later. It was wonderful to have someone who understood what I was going through. It was even more incredible to have a partner who cared about me and supported me through a period of pretty intense anger and self-loathing. I felt dirty. I felt unlovable. I felt unattractive. He helped me get through those feelings, at least temporarily.

It wasn't until I attempted to get back into the dating scene that I realized that not everyone was so understanding. I was rejected countless times. It got to the point that I started disclosing on the first date just to get it over with. My reasoning was at least if (and when) he rejected me, we would have only wasted one date. All those feelings of inadequacy, self-loathing, and depression came flooding back. I became convinced that I was never going to find someone who would want to "deal with" my condition. I felt myself descending into what I have now termed, "the yuck."

The yuck is a place of toxic feelings. It harbors the helpless victim mentality and feeds into feelings of anger, resentment, blame, and sorrow. It is easy to get trapped in the yuck. It's like quicksand. One minute you're doing okay and then as soon as you have a bad date, an outbreak, or even hear a herpes joke, you're right back down in the pit of despair. I felt broken, worthless, and alone.

Gradually, I started to learn more about herpes. I learned about herpes transmission rates and ways to keep outbreaks under control. I learned that there were herpes dating sites and herpes support sites for people with herpes. I found a therapist and did some hard work with her, including letting go of my anger at the guy who raped me (which is how I ended up with herpes). I started to grow. I decided that I needed something to represent my new outlook on life. I'm a firm believer in body reclamation, and for me, that sometimes takes the form of tattoos.

Halloween 2009, three months after the rape that caused the herpes and one month after my herpes diagnosis, I decided to get a lotus tattoo on my right shoulder. The lotus flower grows in the mud in shallow water and does not bloom until it reaches the surface. While it's growing, the flower petals are safe inside the blossom, which keeps them from getting stained by the mud. I always loved the symbolism of the lotus flower, but I didn't realize how accurate the metaphor was for me until about two years later. I battled my anger, my resentment, and my self-consciousness many times over those two years.

Underneath the lotus is a Tibetan Buddhist mantra: "Om Mani Padme Hum." This mantra is a devotion to Avalokiteshvara, the bodhisattva of compassion. It serves as a daily reminder that I cannot know where someone else has been or what has led them to this point. It encourages me to show compassion to others as well as myself.

Healing is not a linear path. There are twists and turns, forks and loops. It took a lot of tears, many sleepless nights, and a lot of support to get me to where I am now. Thanks to my friend Adrial and his wonderful website, the Herpes Opportunity, I found the strength to "come out" about having herpes. I told my friends, family, and the Internet. I have to say, I have never felt so free in my entire life. It feels wonderful to be able to speak openly about having herpes, instead of saying the word in hushed tones while constantly looking over my shoulder wondering who might be listening and judging. I feel genuine and authentic, which is a huge improvement over the way I felt when I was still "in the yuck."

I encourage everyone to take time to reflect on where they are in the growth process. Are you still in the yuck? Don't worry, there are others there too and you can help each other grow. Are you growing but not quite at the surface? Reach out and let people help you. And to those who have blossomed: Share your beauty with the world. Don't be afraid of your roots. Remember them, because they are a testament to your strength and perseverance throughout this journey.

I Was a Teenage Porn Model
Lux Alptraum

I turned eighteen in September 2000. I was a sophomore at Columbia. A lot of significant things happened to me that year: I voted in my first ever election, discovered online dating, launched my first serious relationship, moved into my first real New York City apartment. And in the spring of that year, I began my nude modeling career.

What began as a few striptease photo shoots for a Boston-based website turned into a more ongoing commitment as a cam girl doing weekly cam shows, which later morphed into launching my own indie porn site, perhaps best described as a nerdier, less punk, slightly more hardcore, and far more budget version of Suicide Girls, that had the distinguishing feature of showcasing both male and female models.

In a different version of this story, I stuck with that website, with that career choice, establishing an LA-NYC-SF trifecta with the likes of Joanna Angel and Courtney Trouble (two porn impresarios who began their careers at the same time, under similar circumstances, as I did). But that's not what happened. Instead, at the age of twenty-two, I decided I was sick of it all and shut down my site. I left the world of porn modeling as quickly as I had entered it, and for the most part, I didn't look back.

In recent weeks, award-winning porn director Axel Braun announced that he will no longer work with performers under the age of twenty-one. Braun is not the first to make this decision—almost seven years ago, Oren Cohen's Tightfit Productions made a similar announcement—but as a three-time winner of AVN's Director of the Year award, he may be the most prominent person to eschew working with the under-twenty-one set.

There's a dramatic difference between the mostly softcore photos I modeled for at eighteen and the hardcore features that Braun directs. But as someone who created sexual media at the age of eighteen, I was nonetheless struck by Braun's decision. Would it be better if porn performance were restricted to people over the age of twenty-one? Would I have been better off if I had waited three years before taking my clothes off on camera?

It was hard for me to answer that question, hard even to begin the process of parsing the many emotions it evoked. So I turned to my colleagues in the adult industry to get their thoughts and opinions on the issue.

The first person to respond to me was Bella Vendetta. A dominatrix and porn model whose tastes run towards extreme fetish, Vendetta entered the adult industry at the age of eighteen, training as a dominatrix at the world's oldest BDSM training chateau and shooting her first porn scenes. Three years later, she launched her own fetish site; now, at thirty-two, she's preparing to relaunch the site after a two-year hiatus.

In spite of her own largely positive experiences as a young porn model, Vendetta's views align with Braun's—and then some. In the process of relaunching BellaVendetta.com, she's made the decision to restrict modeling opportunities to those above the age of twenty-five, a full four years older than Braun's age limit.

Why twenty-five? "In my experience young people have a hard time thinking about the rest of their lives," she says. "When you make porn, even if it's just one time, even if it's softcore photos, even if it's for a small website, it will affect you for the rest of your life…. There are certainly some twenty-two-year-old models I know who are incredibly bright and have thought long and hard about the consequences of posing naked on the Internet. But they are few and far between."

There are also her own personal tastes. "I prefer to negotiate scenes with adults…who have enough sexual experience to know what it is they like…. I am not personally turned on by the idea of defiling a young girl."

At nineteen, I spent a few months as a cam model for Ducky Doolittle, a peep-show girl and burlesque performer turned sex educator. Early in our relationship, Doolittle called me to discuss the ramifications of my decision to be naked on the Internet.

"I want to be sure that you know what you're getting into," she said. She wanted to make sure I knew that whatever pictures I modeled for, whatever I publicized, it was forever.

As a younger woman, she'd posed nude for magazines, naïvely thinking that when the month was up and they disappeared from the newsstands, they were gone for good. But nothing ever goes away: people save magazines, images are archived, the choices you make in your youth can always find a way to come back to you as an adult.

As we talked, I told her I understood. I told her I was comfortable with my decision. But over a decade later, I'm not sure that I did, or that I really could. In 2002, it was impossible to predict how the Internet—then a seemingly private, anonymous playground where secrets could live on in the shadows—would mature into a highly public, perpetually archived platform for the mass sharing of information. Whatever I thought I was agreeing to, it wasn't what I actually signed up for.

It's that sort of youthful blindness that's made Vendetta uninterested in working with young models. "I have always made it a policy to fully discuss all the risks of making porn and the ways in which it will affect you forever," she says. "I even put it in my models' contracts that I will not take your photos down if your mom finds out or boyfriend gets mad. But that doesn't stop it from happening.

"When I looked at where these problems were coming from it was always from young models."

In explaining his decision, Braun offered justification for the twenty-one-year minimum thusly: "The percentage of talent who start performing at eighteen and are out of the industry by the time they turn twenty-one is staggering. Those are the ones who are not cut out for porn, and who could very well spend the rest of their lives regretting their choice."

The implication here is clear: porn work should only be pursued by people who plan to make a full-time career out of it. It's a sentiment echoed by Vendetta when she contrasts her experience as a teenage porn performer with that of the young people she's worked with since. "Unlike me, a lot of eighteen- and nineteen-year-olds aren't looking to build an entire career or brand off of the adult industry. They think this sounds fun and crazy and exotic—and the money doesn't hurt either."

It is true that the work you do as an eighteen-year-old porn performer will stick around—and, potentially, haunt you—for the rest of your life. But is that reason enough to limit porn performing to those who aspire to make a career out of it?

Around the time that I was launching my porn website, Courtney Trouble—then an Olympia, WA–based phone-sex operator—was putting together a website known as NoFauxxx (now Indie Porn Revolution). In 2003, Trouble and I connected through message boards and later met in person; we stayed in touch over the years as our careers both diverged and followed parallel paths. These days Trouble lives in Oakland, CA, where she's a part of the vibrant queer porn scene.

Unlike Braun and Vendetta, Trouble isn't convinced that upping the age limit on performing in porn is a good idea—and she doesn't think that leaving the adult industry at twenty-one is necessarily a sign that's one's choice to do sex work was the wrong one.

"A lot of people only do sex work for a few years," she says. "When you're super young it's an incredibly easy way to make money for college or your family or your future plans.

"Leaving the industry quickly doesn't mean it was an age-related mistake. It may actually be more of a reflection on the way that young women are treated in the industry by producers and agents than it is a reflection of their age. If porn were a safer place...maybe [performers would] stick around longer. The question isn't only about age, but labor practices."

★ ★ ★

It is difficult to separate the adult I am today from my decision to pursue porn modeling at the age of eighteen. If I hadn't modeled nude, I wouldn't have fallen in love with the promise of indie porn, and I wouldn't have been inspired to launch my own website—a decision that provided me with the industry knowledge and business sense that later enabled me to take over Fleshbot.

And it's also difficult to deny that, had I waited until twenty-one, I probably wouldn't have ended up on this track. At twenty-one I was out of college, working my first full-time job, and no longer feeling the same thrill I once got from taking off my clothes in front of a camera. At twenty-one, I was ready to move into a more mainstream career. Because as much as I enjoyed making porn, as much as I enjoyed learning about the adult industry, as important as the entire experience was for me, I wasn't interested in being a full-time porn performer. I had never been interested in pursuing porn performance, or porn production, as a full-time, or even long-term, career. At twenty-one, the window of opportunity for experimenting with porn, for experimenting with my identity, was closing. Had I waited until then to model nude, it might have been too late.

Though Trouble isn't convinced that banning teenagers from porn is the best idea, she is encouraged by Braun's attempt to make porn in a more ethical way. "I find it encouraging that mainstream porn directors are trying to find ways to bring their own ethics to their work. Each of us as directors experience the industry differently because we all make different movies, and maybe for Axel—taking advantage of brand-new adults isn't something he wants to risk doing."

Age restrictions are certainly one way to attempt a more

ethical porn-production environment. But it seems worth wondering whether there are other ways to ensure that everyone on a porn set is safe, respected, and taken care of, rather than merely limiting performance to those presumably old enough to know how to advocate for themselves.

I shuttered my porn site at twenty-two, and quit the adult industry completely a few months later. I thought I was done with the whole thing, and even when I found myself reimmersed in the world of porn through my work at Fleshbot, I still couldn't imagine myself jumping back into the fray and attempting to be a model or a performer. And then, at twenty-nine, I did another nude photo shoot. I was in Toronto for the Feminist Porn Awards, sharing a hotel room with Courtney Trouble and Jiz Lee, a talented and respected genderqueer porn performer. In the bathroom, Lee and I stripped down and took a bubble bath together, drinking champagne out of tiny, single-serving bottles, and we giggled and made out and played in the tub. Trouble photographed us, and the pictures ended up showcased on Karma Pervs, Lee's philanthropic porn project. At twenty-nine, in a porn-friendly career, on a set with my friends, there was nothing dangerous or threatening about being naked in front of a camera. I didn't have to worry about who might find the photos, I didn't have to worry about the effect they might have on my career. I could enjoy myself and simply celebrate the experience of being a sexual person, making sexual art.

Most people don't have the freedom that I had that day. Most people—especially young people—can't dip in and out of the sex industry without worrying about the blemish it might place on their résumé, the damage it might do to their relationships.

But perhaps if they did, we wouldn't have to worry so much about whether every eighteen-year-old who wants to shoot a porn scene is going to still be doing porn five, or ten, or twenty years down the line. If it was easier to shift between the worlds of porn work and mainstream work—to dip your toes in the adult industry without fear of permanently ruining your résumé—then teenagers intrigued by the adult industry could have the freedom to experiment with it without being burdened to commit to it. Teenagers could have the freedom to be teenagers, without fear of permanently blemishing their future.

But failing that, maybe limiting teenagers' involvement in porn isn't the worst thing. If involvement in sexual media is destined to be a life-altering choice, it's one that should be made by people old enough to understand the ramifications of that.

Disability and Sex
Jason Armstrong

After two pot brownies, my friend Alex was in fine form at the party we were at. Minus the pot brownies, this was a pretty staid group of people, but once Alex got a little high, all bets were off. "You're so attractive. You make me moist!" he bellowed at some mortified straight man. My head spun only to find Alex talking to said straight man and his girlfriend. Alex was propositioning them for a threesome but qualified it to the girl by saying it was only to get into her boyfriend's pants. I decided the straight couple needed to be rescued from Alex and went over. "You'll have to excuse Alex, he's had a stroke, and he's had two brownies."

"The stroke didn't take away my sight and I know an attractive man when I see one," Alex said, taking one more glance at the straight man as I pulled him away. "Do you want to sniff my diaper?"

Alex was indeed wearing a diaper, and was just the kind of man who let everybody know it. It was a badge of honor for all that he had been through. He'd already been living with HIV since the early '80s, since before HIV had a name. His bowels and bladder didn't always give him much warning. I remember the day I received a call from our mutual friend David in September, telling me that Alex had had a stroke and was in the emergency room at the General.

I got to the hospital and found Alex. The right side of his body was paralyzed, including his face. His mouth drooped on the right side and his speech was slurred. He looked up at me as I knelt to kiss his forehead. "They say I might not ever walk again," he said, enunciating as best he could.

"We'll get through this Alex. You'll walk again, I know it," I countered.

"Damn right I'll walk again. There are still men to fuck."

Alex didn't see the inside of his apartment again for four long months. After being in the emergency room for a torturous week until they could find him a room, and then two weeks in that hospital room, he was transferred to a rehabilitation center. While I watered the plants in Alex's apartment and collected his mail, Alex engaged in the arduous task of learning to use the right side of his body. His doctors warned that another stroke was not an impossibility. He battled through and was released from the rehab center just before Christmas. And that's when he completely broke down.

Alex was henceforth differently-abled, if you will. He required a brace to walk, to walk ever so carefully. His right arm was still immobile. We had dinner together every Saturday night once he returned home. We would order pizza and I would read the latest essay I'd written for my sex blog to him. He was the one person to hear my essays before I posted them, and my short essay would launch us into an examination of our sex lives. Alex never allowed for bitterness, but I remember the Saturday night that he looked at me and asked, with tears in his eyes, "Will a man ever want to be with me again?"

I remembered, long ago, in my midtwenties, being at the New York City Pride Parade. I recall only two moments from that parade, and both of them left a deep impression on the young gay man that I was. The first moment was when the float passed by on which there were men who had fought at Stonewall on that fateful night in '69, when our history changed forever. These men were old, with canes and in wheelchairs. They had been there, and they were here with us now. As they floated down the street, I realized I'd just witnessed history. My history. The whooping from the crowd told me that everyone around me was sharing the exact same feeling.

The second moment that I recall was when a gay group in wheelchairs passed by. Young and old, of every race, their presence hit me. It became all too clear, all at once, that our society neglects to recognize the disabled as sexual. And here they were, claiming their orientation, refusing to be left in the shadows or on the sidelines. As with the men who had fought at Stonewall, I knew I was witnessing something that I did not feel much of within my own belly: I was witnessing what looked like courage, and I found it beautiful.

After Alex had his stroke, I did some research—on Xtube. I found an instructional video for sex workers on how to best cater to the needs of their disabled clientele. And then I found a video by a man who suffered from some type of palsy. He was jacking off and I so wanted to be there with him. His pits, his cock, his absolute engagement were hot—his palsy did not matter. I wrote him a message telling him how amazing his video was and posted a comment on his profile. I didn't hear back from him.

Alex is improving. He's walking without a brace, and he's getting movement back in his right arm and hand. He's even venturing forth to the Eagle again. More than that, he got picked up recently and took the man back to his place. But he called me to tell me that it didn't work. His body did not want to cooperate with his desire. He was momentarily bereft. He is not supposed to take Viagra, but to hell with it—he ordered some online and his doctor is turning a blind eye for him. Alex is a force to be reckoned with.

Last night, I hit the streets of the Village to go get a pack of cancer-causing smokes. I began to think about the ways we are all disabled. For some of us, it is visible to others. But for many, it's invisible. It's the disease that's eating us from the inside. It's the mental anguish that we mask so as to appear normal. Among the many casualties of illness or disability is our sexuality. Always, we are fighting to reclaim it, from external forces, or internal.

As I walked down the steps from the tobacco shop, I noticed a young man in a motorized wheelchair. He couldn't have been more than twenty-four. He, like the man in the Xtube video I had watched, appeared to suffer from a palsy. He was alone on the street, in this Gay Village, and he looked bewildered, lost. He did not see me see him. And he was gorgeous. My instinct was to reach out to him. I wanted to make love to him. I wanted to let him know that if he was in the Village seeking comfort from the men who walked by, he would find it. I wanted to take his cock in my mouth. I wanted to enter him and fill him with light so that he shone like a nuclear reactor. I wanted to believe that my feelings were not born of pity or fear that by the grace of god, that could be me. I wanted to apologize to him if these thoughts were in any way construed as condescending or patronizing. I wanted to tell him that even though I am so-called able-bodied, I have struggled since childhood with an illness that I rarely discuss, an illness that constantly thwarts my sexuality, an illness that no one can see, but that I experience so profoundly. I wanted... But instead, seeing him carry on down the sidewalk, I too continued on my way. But oh how I wanted...

When Alex first got home from rehab, he was sternly warned against walking too far from home. And to walk, especially in the beginning, was laborious for Alex. But secretly, one day, Alex walked from his apartment to the nearest tattoo parlor. The next Saturday night, he surprised with me his tattoo. On the inside of his left forearm, he'd had the word Courage inscribed in glorious script. I wondered, like the Cowardly Lion from *The Wizard of Oz*, if I would ever have the courage to both come back from an illness, or to even get and stay sick, and still reclaim myself and my sexuality. In my twenties, I thought that the perfect man was the one with the six-pack abs. But Alex's courage to face disability and still move forward changed that. I think that having just turned forty, I am maybe, just maybe, growing up.

Fumbling Towards Humanity: How "Trans Grrrls" Helped Me Open Up to My Partner
Amy Dentata

I was single by choice for years before I felt the dating itch again. I took to OKcupid and, on the rare occasion someone actually responded, met up with a stranger. Without fail, we would realize we lacked chemistry and never see each other again. After each dating failure, I felt a mixture of sadness and relief. A failed date meant I didn't have to worry about physical intimacy. It meant I didn't have to worry about taking my clothes off in front of another person. It meant I didn't have to face the chance of, at best, another Teachable Moment regarding transphobia, or at worst, mortal danger.

I lose no matter what. Giving cis partners the Trans 101 talk is exhausting. When dating other trans people, I still feel gross because of my body. I'm pre-op and very uncomfortable about my genitalia. It's hard for me to get off even just masturbating. I have to cover myself in blankets and touch myself just right so my anatomy feels like it's configured the right way. Sometimes I'm okay using my current equipment, but even then it feels weird. It's just weird in a way I can enjoy. At least when masturbation does work, I know exactly what buttons to push. I know just the right way to jiggle the door handle, the right twist to turn on the faucet. Teaching that to someone else takes time. It requires a partner who is willing to listen, and who can handle freakouts when my body upsets me. The stars have to align just right to find a partner like that. Dating is a crapshoot for anybody, but for me the odds are stacked even higher.

The stars did align recently, though. I'm seeing someone new, a wonderful cis girl I will call Kate. (Disclosure: even though I exclude identifying information, I asked her permission before writing this article, as it includes personal details of our sexy times.) In Kate I found a partner who not only thinks I'm sexy, but understands my body issues, and is willing to learn all the quirks involved in getting me off.

Our first physical exploration involved cuddling. Cuddling is amazing with her. It usually takes a long time for me to warm up, but with her I get turned on almost immediately. Once I try to move beyond cuddling, however, I freeze. My first time with her, I was reluctant to take off my clothes. I was scared of rejection and felt mortified about my body. I also felt alone. Profoundly alone, in a way that's hard to describe.

Cisgender people have representation everywhere in the media. Images of them dating, making out, and getting dirty are on TV, movies, books, commercials, billboards, just about everywhere. Mainstream representation of women like me, on the other hand, is rare and usually follows a predictable script: cis man unwittingly goes out with trans woman, cis man finds out she's trans (always in the form of a joke at the woman's expense), cis man vomits and/or kills her.

There is no romance for trans women in the media unless the plot involves a tragic ending. We are either a punch line or a Very Special Episode of "Blossom." We can't just fall in love, get in normal fights, have hot makeup sex, or any other romantic activity cis people take for granted. In mainstream porn, we are made into fantasy creatures that exist only to fulfill the taboo fantasies of cisgender straight men. There aren't widely known cultural stories and dating norms that include trans women. We are always on the frontier, and while that can feel exhilarating, it's also alienating.

The first time Kate and I had sex, I was too nervous to orgasm. It wasn't for lack of support, either. She was a caring, listening lover. She eagerly learned the ways I like being touched, and what to avoid so I don't get dysphoric. Our second time together, as I reached the same impassable plateau, I asked her to stop, and lay there crying. Dysphoria and anti-trans baggage won out. I felt disgusting. She wished she could do something to help. We sat on the bed and chatted for a while. To pass the time, I showed her my strap-on harness and my porn DVDs. *Trans Grrrls* in particular caught her eye. As the night ended she reassured me, "You don't have to apologize." For anything: for my body issues, for crying, for feeling insecure.

Kate and I fell headfirst into the infatuation phase of our relationship. The next day during work, she told me over Facebook that she was reading through my blog, because she just couldn't get enough of me. That scared me, because I've written a lot about my dating frustrations as a trans woman, and the ways cis people have hurt me. Would she get offended by me talking about cis people in a negative light? Would she think I'm too angry? I was convinced she would find a reason somewhere in my blog to hate me. But she still made plans for our next date. This time, I was sleeping over.

At her place we cuddled and immediately got turned on, like our previous times together. It was our third time together in the sheets, and my anxiety levels were increasing with each encounter. Surely, that night my transness would ruin everything. I was too broken and strange for anyone to love.

"You wanted to watch one of my DVDs, right?" I asked. I'd brought several, but out came *Trans Grrrls*, the subject on the tip of both our tongues. We lay together, bodies wrapped around each other, and watched the opening scene with Chelsea Poe and Maxine Holloway.

"That place looks familiar," she said.

"They filmed the opening part at the Dyke March last year." We both lamented having missed the march.

"It's so hot that they're actually doing it right there in public," she said. I agreed, mostly by moaning, because at that point her hands were traveling all over me.

Then the scene cut to an apartment, and Chelsea and Maxine tore off each other's clothes. There on the screen was someone like me, having sex with someone like Kate. They were both happy, enthusiastic, and into each other. No "surprise reveal," no horrified reaction shots, no cis gaze ruminating on how a trans partner might affect a cis person's feelings about their sexual orientation. Just two women fucking.

It made me feel human. And naked, even though my clothes were already off. A layer of psychic armor hardened by slurs, stereotypes, and violence melted off my body. It felt like the universe said to me, "We have a place for you. You belong here."

I said to Kate, "In a little bit you're going to find out something

I love about Maxine." Maxine laughs when she comes, and it is so adorable. Kate agreed. Sometime after the second scene of the film, I had an amazing orgasm, all thanks to Kate. The isolation I felt during our previous encounters washed away. That orgasm was a revelation, a moment of healing, and I laughed like Maxine through the intense torrent of emotions. That was the first time I've ever laughed while coming instead of crying.

I regret to say I had a hard time paying attention to the rest of the film. By the end of the night I was completely exhausted, in the best way possible. I didn't think the evening would end with me lying in bed with her, catching my breath, but there we were.

"I read in your blog that cis women scare you," she said. Oh no. The exact words in my blog were, "Cis women scare the shit out of me." Their bodies make me feel inferior, masculine, fake. Their mere presence can feel like it's erasing my identity.

"Yeah," I said, hiding my face in her boobs like I'd suddenly forgotten object permanence.

"Does that mean I scare you too?"

"Sometimes." I didn't want to say it, but I wasn't going to lie.

She was supposed to get offended. Supposed to say, "We're not ALL like that, you know!" Supposed to dismiss my problems as whiny hypersensitivity, like countless people before her. Instead, she cooed and petted my hair. She said that hopefully she can be less scary. She kept holding me. She wouldn't let go, and I didn't want her to. I belonged there.

In Defense of Celibacy
Lauren Marie Fleming
aka Queerie Bradshaw

Celibacy is underrated.

This statement may sound hypocritical coming from a person who makes her living writing about the antithesis of abstinence, but my life is often controlled by sex, so I understand the importance of taking time away from it and focusing on other things.

Like learning to play bridge. Or crocheting. Or, you know, actually dealing with the fact that you watched your brother bleed out and die in front of you.

Shit like that.

There's something to be said for taking sexual energy and aiming it somewhere else. Queen Elizabeth, Joan of Arc, Florence Nightingale, these women put their sexual frustration to good use. I'm not looking to run a country or fight a holy war, but I bet I'd finally finish my memoir about sex if I quit spending so much time having it.

Monks and priests have been known to levitate, survive being set on fire, and heal the dying. Give up sex and all that extra energy can go into performing unbelievable feats. Just last week, instead of going on the two dates I had planned, I cleaned my whole apartment, washed every article of clothing I owned and neatly organized my extensive sex toy collection: a bona fide miracle.

Like most lesbians, I've dabbled in hippy, new-age, touchy-feely emotional exploration, but as much as I love a good drum circle beating out Ani DiFranco's greatest hits, I'm more of the in a dungeon beating on a stranger type.

Or I was.

Now I don't really know who I am and what I want. Two years ago this week, my sister and her baby came horribly close to dying during premature labor. A month later, my brother was diagnosed with cancer. A month after that, my grandmother had a stroke at my law school graduation. Ten days later, I watched her die. About once a month after that, my brother had some tumor removed from or poison put into his body. Then he had his jaw removed. Then a month later, I watched him die.

After that, all I wanted to do was get drunk, fuck, and shoot guns, so that is what I did.

Then my grandfather, Poppo, one of the most important people in my life, a man who shared my birthday and taught me to paint, died. For the last week of his life, I helped feed him morphine, sang him songs and held his hand, watching the light slowly fade from his loving eyes.

Soon, we were planning yet another funeral, the third for my family in eighteen months and nothing could be said or done to make me feel better. Including sex. Instead, the thing I love to do most in the world has become a chore, yet another emotionally painful thing to endure.

The vulnerability that having sex caused in me was destroying me and I was destroying any chance of a solid, healthy relationship with someone in return.

It was time to be consciously celibate, to take sex, and the horrible insecurities it now caused in me, out of the equation.

This realization scared me. We live in a sex-dominated culture and I make my living being right there in the heart of it, experiencing every bit I can and sharing my findings. I've engaged in a plethora of pleasure for the sake of a good story. I go for the risqué and raunchy because it gives good headline.

It's hard to purposely give that up, but give it up I am, until June 6, the day my completed memoir is due.

I'm still going to attend all the porn conventions, sex worker get-togethers, BDSM play parties, dominatrix gang bangs and tantric workshops I have planned between now and June 6, I'm just not going to be quite as participatory.

I almost didn't say anything to anyone, but then Jenn, an amazing radical, fat, femme blogger colleague of mine reminded me that, "Intentionally not engaging in partnered sex is political and complicated and worth talking about."

So here I am, a kinky queer sex writer, making a statement by not having sex.

I'm not quite sure what that statement's going to look like yet; first I have to figure out what exactly I'm giving up, what celibacy means to me. One of my closest friends gives up sex all the time, taking vows of celibacy from hours to months depending on what he's looking to accomplish in his life at that moment. His celibacy attempts to delete all sexual thoughts from his mind and therefore masturbating is not allowed.

When he asked me if I would do the same, I replied, "I'm a not a fuckin' saint here." However, as I think about it, if finishing my memoir and writing more is one of my goals, I may have to give up masturbating as well. I spend (sometimes waste) a big portion of my days reviewing sex toys and porn over and over again, you know, for work. If I gave that up, or limited it at least, I'd have a lot more time to work on projects that pay my bills.

But who am I kidding, I'm not Joan of Arc. I haven't gone a week without masturbating since I discovered the joy of a vibrating toy at age six. Masturbation is staying on the table.

Romantic dates, however, are off the table. Way too time consuming, trying to get to know someone new. If I want dinner, I have to call a friend. Penetration is obviously off, including any oral sex, but I'm going to play kissing, cuddling and nonsexual BDSM interactions by ear.

I feel like I'm missing something, but all I can think about is fisting.

This may be more difficult than anticipated.

I once took a vow of celibacy for two months after a bad split from a long-term relationship. About two weeks into it, I was heading to go break that vow when I broke my foot and ankle instead.

I don't believe in a vengeful God judging from above, but I still feel like he was punishing me for my sins that night, angry at me for attempting to break my promise to myself. If thinking about having sex caused a cast, I'm worried about ending in full-body traction if I fuck up this new vow.

It always seems like the minute I decide to stop looking for sex, sex comes looking for me. I've had three offers in the two days since I made the decision to take a break from sex, all from people I really want inside of me. I'm currently writing this sitting at a house on the beach in a bikini next to a hot butch, who is testing my resolve by looking quite dapper in an outfit set for captaining our invisible yacht.

It's harder than it sounds, to not have sex. To not reach over, grab his hand and lead him to the back room, or better yet wait a few hours until it's dark and lead us to the shoreline, waves crashing our bodies together.

When your brain is constantly an erotica novel, it's really hard to not act out these fantasies.

Sure, the butch and I are just here as friends, simply enjoying a sunny San Diego day together, but I know how good he feels against me, I know exactly what I'm missing out on.

Unfortunately, that includes emotional instability right now as well. I haven't felt this way about someone in a very long time, but I changed that moment I saw my brother die and now I have no idea what I want from sex or a relationship, making navigating both impossible.

Once I gave up sex with the person I was seeing (and liked) the most, it was surprisingly easy to give up the others, sending them back into friend zones, explaining to them that I'm just not there right now, that too many funerals have left me with no energy for sex, no ability to be vulnerable in yet another way. It was shockingly simple.

At first.

Now I want to hump everything that moves, rotates or vibrates in any way. If I'm going to be serious about this temporary break from sex, I'm going to need help, so naturally I turned to Twitter and Facebook for advice. Soon my inbox was flooded with stories from my amazing followers of what they did, learned and changed through consciously and purposely abstaining from sex.

I started with the stories from people who, like me, quit having sex because their grief was too overwhelming. A woman who first met me through my online dating profile explained why she quit having sex after her father and friend died close together:

"I didn't feel inclined to share any part of me with any other person.... I'd worked so hard to put all of my pieces back together, and I was afraid that if I let anybody in, they'd just shake those pieces loose and I'd be a crumbling mess again. My abstinence acted as my mortar for a strong foundation."

The theme of building a solid emotional foundation through abstaining from sex was present in almost every story I read. In a society with an arguably unhealthy obsession for quick pleasure, it's not surprising people would feel a need to give up sex to feel emotionally stable, fulfilled even.

There are times in your life when a quick fuck can be beneficial, but sometimes all sex does is add to the confusion that is life. Sex with others muddies the emotional waters; take sex away and there's a better chance of finding clarity within yourself.

"I spent approximately four years without having sex during my mid-20s. At the time I was sure I shouldn't be dating vanilla girls, and I did explore the possibility that I am gay because of my cross-dressing and pegging desires. It took me a while to both realize and accept that I am a sissy who needs a naturally dominant female, and those years of not having sex helped me by avoiding further confusion of trying to be something I'm not with the wrong women.

Once I realized what I needed, I sought it, found it, and am happier than I've ever been.... I attribute much of this to those years I had to discover myself."

This story from a Twitter follower of mine reminded me that I'm not new to the act of abstaining. After bad and boring sex with men in high school, I didn't have sex for three years. I had absolutely no interest in it, which was sad and shocking to me at the time, until I had sex with a woman and WHOA, there's what I was missing.

Counting up all the periods of abstaining from sex, both consciously and consequentially, one-third of my sexual life has been marked by a lack of the act. Looking back, those were the most productive years of my life. They were also the most lonely ones as well. There has to be a balance, but I've yet to find it, and when faced with sex or sleep, I choose the latter, which is why I'm single but my skin is fabulous.

One thing I've learned is that there's a detox period and it gets easier with time. It's not that you forget what you're missing, you just learn to live without it consuming you. I'm not alone in this feeling. A Twitter follower of mine wrote:

"If I've learned anything from not being active for a while it's that sex just really isn't that important to me in the long run, especially if I'm not dating anyone. I have a friend who dates regularly and has a rolodex of partners to choose from. She has an active sex life and is used to it. She recently visited her parents for a week and upon her return she was almost frantic from not having any while she was gone.... I enjoy sex and all, but I've never understood the physical craving for it that (I suppose) comes from engaging in it regularly."

I understand that craving all too well. I've understood that craving since I was six. I explore that craving religiously, both personally and professionally.

I've never been one for religions with puritanical teachings, never thought of pleasure as a bad thing, but I'm learning to respect religious people who abstain for their own emotional and physical benefit.

Jenny, a blogger buddy of mine, wrote to me about her choice to find herself and God during her self-induced abstinence period:

"It was hard at first...but when I got accustomed to it, there was actually a lot of freedom in it. When I met a guy at an event, through a mutual friend, or at church, there was never that thought of 'what will he think of me?' and a tendency to perform as there had been in the past."

Maybe that's what it is, maybe I'm just tired of performing, pretending I'm okay when I'm really not, feeling especially like I have to be okay with sex, the thing in which I am a supposed expert. The question "How are you doing?" is impossible for me to honestly answer these days because I have no clue how I am doing; I haven't even begun to figure that out.

As much as I wish sex were the answer, it's becoming glaringly apparent that it's not. It helped at first, letting my grief give way to pleasure, shutting off and shutting out, but eventually I imploded on myself and now I'm even messier than before.

I'm not sure what this break will accomplish. I'm not even sure what I'm looking to get out of this sexless period. But I do know that I already feel a weight lifted from my shoulders at knowing I can guiltlessly stay in and write Wednesday instead of going to the local lesbian night to try to get laid.

No Restrictions
Dee Dee Behind

My very first session with a client with severe disabilities was while I was working as a professional dominatrix on the third floor of a dungeon in an elevator-less building. In addition to the logistical nightmare of getting a man in a motorized wheelchair onto four hours of public transportation and then up three flights of stairs, how, exactly, was I to tie up someone who was already completely physically immobile?

Paul, a man in his fifties with a degenerative condition that affected his nervous system, wrote a letter, a snail-mail letter, to the listed PO box of the dungeon, explaining his deep and unrelenting desire to be whipped. This, he said, had captured his imagination ever since our dungeon was featured on a silly public access television show that highlights the "wild and offbeat" places of my hometown of Chicago.

Paul explained in his nearly illegible and deliberate handwriting his concern that his parents, still his primary caregivers despite his own age and independence, might think he was being abused by his attendants should they find marks or bruises on his body. He was deeply ashamed to admit that this had happened in the past after he managed to pinch his own genitals for sexual pleasure until he left deep purple bruises. The suspected attendant had been fired and was barely spared criminal charges, and Paul would never live down the regret he felt for the trouble he caused her.

But to come clean and discuss desire, particularly his pleasure in pain, was not an option for him. It was one thing to have erections during sponge baths, but a penchant for masochism would have been too much for those who cared for him. Paul was surrounded by people whom he depended on, not just for a lifeline to all things physically beyond the reach of his crippled body, but also for their emotional ties to him created by his own helplessness. His helplessness was his survival.

As a sex worker, I can imagine that if the source of those bruises were traced back to me, the consequences would be devastating. It freaks me out right now, just thinking about it. I imagine how I might explain consent to reporters at my courthouse interview while standing trial for felony sexual abuse of the helplessly disabled. How could consent exist in such a lopsided power dynamic? To believe that this was a consensual sexual experience would mean to concede to the sexual autonomy of a man who cannot feed or clothe himself. But here were the man's desires, in black smudgy ink, an eloquent request he preferred to submit to me in writing, because, as the letter continued to explain, his ability to speak is also severely impaired and therefore he is unable to express himself with speech. Great. I imagined myself burning in hell in fishnets.

After Paul arrived in his motorized wheelchair, and a long

battle to get him up the stairs in the chair failed, I chained up the chair with my bicycle lock to the steel handles of our downstairs lobby doors, while the house wrestling domme carried him up the three flights of stairs to the dungeon. After strapping him to a wheeling gurney we kept as a medical prop in the "doctor's office," I carefully undressed him. I was terrified I was going to hurt him. The irony.

Paul's body was twisted and unwieldy, his skin a pasty white. His bony apple-shaped rib cage was topped with a huge lopsided head, giving it the illusion of growing out of his shoulder. His face was frozen in an insane smile. I could not tell if he was incredibly happy or horribly contorted. I peeled down his pants to discover, to my nineteen-year-old only-a-year-in-the-biz shock, a raging-hard penis, prominent and quite impressive in size. It stuck straight out of the dark recess of his lap, a lap permanently frozen in a sitting position.

He made little encouraging snorting noises as I admonished him for being a horny little slut—so encouraging in fact, that I raised my hand in a threatening gesture as if I were going to slap his cock in punishment for his digressions. When I did this, Paul went wild. His eyes grew huge and he spasmed with excitement, making these crazy disturbing honking noises that emanated deep from inside his face. The entire session was one long negotiation of me being terrified I was hurting him, and him getting incredibly turned on, and then me becoming a little less terrified, and on and on it went. In the end, he came multiple times with only the stimulation of a riding crop whipping his cock—the mark of a true masochist.

After hauling wheelchairs up and down flights of stairs more than once in the past fifteen years of being a sex worker, I think about the barriers to sexual pleasure people who are disabled face all the time, both the physical and the social. In addition to the isolation people with disabilities face, stemming from their exclusion from physical spaces and communities designed for able-bodied adults only, many social situations prohibit people with disabilities from fully participating in their own sexuality. The world continues to shift and change around disability, but sexuality seems the exemption.

However, despite being shielded most of their lives from the topic of sexuality, no disabled client has ever contacted me with the naïveté about sex that is portrayed in Hollywood versions of disability. Portrayals of sexuality of the disabled as innocent assuage our discomfort around the topic of different bodies and queerness. The reason they "feel good" is because they confront what disturbs us about the desires of the non-desirable. Their sexuality is transformed into something normative and comfortable only if we recast the disabled as children, and the hookers as saints.

A few years ago, I received an email from Justin, a twenty-two-year-old virgin. He explained he was a person with a disease that made him unable to use his muscles and therefore needed a wheelchair, constant care, and an attendant who was typing the very email that I was presently reading. He was a virgin, and could I help him? He had the blessing of his attendant, but not his disapproving parents, who still spoke to him in a baby voice. Could I accommodate the unusual situation?

I squinted to examine the picture attached to the email, showing a face propped up with pillows inside a huge motorized chair that swallowed his tiny frame. The idea of taking something—anything—from him made me feel uncomfortable.

I knew that stigmatization of disability was the real barrier to Justin's sexual satisfaction, not his inability to use his limbs. By recognizing my own feelings of discomfort as an acculturation to infantilize Justin, and responding to him instead as the horny twenty-two-year-old he was, I was trying to practice direct resistance to the everyday sexual oppressions and stigmas that all queer-bodied people face. Part of why I love being a sex worker is because I am part of a revolution to liberate the world from shame, heteronormativity, and social isolation.

But, at the same time, I grew up on this planet the same as everyone else. I try to unpack my privilege, and sometimes I fall short: I hate my girl body, I "yuck" someone's "yum," or I am too scared to touch twisted limbs. Even though I'm scared, I keep chipping away at my own shit, going deeper and deeper into that world of Balls-Out Whore Fantastica, where everyone wears leopard-print spandex and speaks openly and curiously about shocking topics at the dinner table. This is how we get that way, that place where the shocking is normal. Among other things, it is one of the sex-worker superpowers that makes us soldiers in this revolution; we pull it together and pretend someone didn't just scare the shit out of us with their drunken violence, that they didn't just shit in our hand, or they didn't deeply offend us with a stigmatizing backhanded compliment mid-fellatio. Or, at the very least, that all these things happened, but didn't bother us one bit.

I didn't offer Justin any special accommodation except to waive my extra hundred-dollar travel fee. Is this a practice that balances helpful but not patronizing? To respect his sexuality by treating him like any other man, even if that means shaking him down for all he's got? Is charging full price an act of solidarity? Or am I risking blowing his cover, because honestly, this man has no job, and how the hell can he hide a three-hundred-dollar bank account withdrawal? Did Justin feel like he had a political ally in this sex worker, someone who could provide comfort in his sexual normalcy, as I do for all of my clients? Or am I just a blood-sucking whore to him too? After all, he grew up on the same planet as everyone else.

He and his attendant conspired to use the attendant's father's house while he was away on vacation, making the appointment an all-day production and a complex web of deceit for both of them. For me, it was a 2:00 p.m. outcall. I borrowed the car of a friend, another sex worker.

"I'm leaving now!" I yelled, picking up the keys from her foyer table. My friend in her computer room-slash-home office-slash-webcamming stage didn't answer. "Going to take a crippled man's vir-gin-it-yyyy," I singsonged, pausing for an answer from down the hall.

"Have fun," she said, without even directing her voice towards the door to the hallway.

"You're so amazing," said a voice off the foyer, just as I was opening the front door. I turned and it was my friend's roommate. Leaning against the kitchen counter with a cup of tea in both hands, she cocked her head and made a face. I know this face. It's the "sex work is a public service" face. It's the "you are such a good person...and I could never do what you do" face. For the first time since booking this session, I felt gross. I wanted to scratch her eyes out.

I drove around a deserted subdivision looking for the address number along rows of identical-looking houses. I found the house because it was the only one with a car in the driveway—an ancient gray minivan covered in special designation stickers, yellow warnings on all sides, and bulky door modifications, sitting in all its disabled obviousness in the driveway.

When I knocked on the door, I was surprised to find that the attendant, a profession usually reserved for women, was instead a handsome young frat boy about Justin's age. He explained that

Justin wanted to skip through the undignified aspect of making me wait the thirty minutes it took to get him from clothed in a wheelchair to naked in bed, so they did it already. Justin was waiting in the bedroom, and he hoped I wasn't freaked out. "I'm not," I lied.

In a whisper, the attendant expressed his ambivalence about helping Justin get laid, since he could lose his job, or possibly worse. He was visibly distraught describing how no one around him took Justin seriously as a young man, not just censoring him from the world of adults, but also disallowing him the right to grow up.

He feared Justin's parents were emotionally invested in keeping Justin five years old. He was afraid that by denying Justin his desire to finally get laid, he would be just like the parents. So he consented to help, even though he really didn't want to. After some consoling and reassurance, I was led to the doors of the bedroom. I slipped though the double doors alone, into the dark, carpeted chamber. The bed consumed the entire room. At first I didn't see him, his small body covered in folds of sheets. But my eyes adjusted, and from the doorway, I could make out the side of his face, his hair, a shoulder, all completely still.

"Justin?" I said, into the quiet.

Without moving or laying eyes on me, he bellowed, "Hello there, sexy!"

My session with Justin was unremarkable in that when it came right down to it, Justin was like any other man who is twenty-two and still a virgin—wide-eyed and easy to impress. Justin was mature, funny, and self-deprecating, and I enjoyed his company, careful to not lay the hustle on too thick, lest he mistake my desire to make him feel good for the paternalism that is suspiciously heaped onto people with disabilities. Able-bodied men, hilariously enough, have no such "bullshit meter" for praise.

I imagine Justin had a great time, but I doubt he could care less about the intersecting politics of disability and sex work. He was, after all, just wanting to get laid out of the arrangement, and wasn't really interested in joining a whore revolution. And I, for all my radical political beliefs, am in this game to get paid. I like to think something is traded in those exchanges besides sex and money, but you never really know. I know that I made some kind of impression on Justin, because I got an email from him a week later. Thanks for the good time, he said, but I am not his type. Did I have a friend? Someone blonde perhaps, with big breasts?

About the Authors

LAURA AGUSTÍN (The Naked Anthropologist at lauraagustin. com) is an authority on undocumented migration and commercial sex. Her book *Sex at the Margins: Migration, Labour Markets and the Rescue Industry* shows how prostitution is isolated as a feminist debate and how moral crusaders use neocolonialist ideas of deviance and crime to repress migration and infantilize women.

LUX ALPTRAUM is a writer, sex educator and consultant specializing in sex technology. Past projects have included gigs as the editor, publisher and CEO of Fleshbot; a sex educator at an adolescent pregnancy prevention program; an HIV pretest counselor; and the founder of ThatStrangeGirl, an alternative porn site, and Boinkology.

JASON ARMSTRONG is the author of the blog Hunting for

Sex: Cautionary Tales from the Quest (huntingforsex.blogspot. ca), voted by Kinkly.com as one of the top 100 sex blogs on the net. Jason is currently working on his first book, entitled *Gooning: Portrait of a Masturbator.*

DEE DEE BEHIND is a sex worker, mostly. She wrote her piece in a writing class at her fancy Ivy League university. On the last day of class, after workshopping her story to her shocked peers, a fellow classmate approached her in the hallway. "I'm a sex worker, too," she grinned.

RACHEL KRAMER BUSSEL (rachelkramerbussel.com) is the author of *Sex & Cupcakes: A Juicy Collection of Essays* and a sex columnist for *Philadelphia City Paper* and *DAME.* She teaches erotic writing workshops at colleges, conferences, sex toy stores and online, and has edited over fifty anthologies such as *The Big Book of Orgasms.*

LYNN COMELLA, PHD is an Associate Professor of Gender and Sexuality Studies at the University of Nevada, Las Vegas. She writes a regular column on sexuality and culture for *Vegas Seven* magazine, and is co-editor (with Shira Tarrant) of the book *New Views on Pornography: Sexuality, Politics, and the Law.*

AMY DENTATA (amydentata.com) is a writer, game designer and performer whose writing has appeared on Autostraddle and in *Trans Bodies, Trans Selves,* a resource guide for the trans community, and in her self-published chapbook, *Bite.* She has also spoken about trans issues at colleges across the U.S.

EPIPHORA (HeyEpiphora.com) has been testing sex toys and writing about them on her blog for seven years. She has been featured in VICE, Playboy *XBIZ Premiere* magazine and Tristan Taormino's *The Secrets of Great G-Spot Orgasms and Female Ejaculation*, but her greatest accomplishment is that readers entrust their future orgasms to her.

LAUREN MARIE FLEMING (LaurenMarieFleming.com) is a writer and motivator who believes in radical self-love, mind-blowing sex and the healing power of writing. Formerly known as Queerie Bradshaw, Lauren is the founder of the Frisky Feminist Collective & Press (FriskyFeminist.com), and creator of the Bawdy Love movement (BawdyLove.com).

ALEXANDRIA GODDARD has over twenty-five years of combined experience in legal investigations, fraud/risk management investigations and social media analysis. She has appeared on shows such as "Dr. Phil," "20/20," "Piers Morgan," "Democracy Now," "Jane Velez-Mitchell" and in a multitude of print and web-based articles regarding the Steubenville, Ohio rape case.

FIONA HELMSLEY's writing can be found in various anthologies like *Ladyland* and *Air in the Paragraph Line* and online at websites like Jezebel, Junk Lit, The Hairpin and The Rumpus. Her book of essays, stories and poems, *My Body Would be the Kindest of Strangers* is forthcoming in 2015.

TINA HORN produces and hosts "Why Are People Into That?!", a podcast that demystifies desire. She holds an MFA in Creative Nonfiction Writing from Sarah Lawrence College. Her first book, *Love Not Given Lightly*, is a collection of nonfiction stories about sex workers.

MITCH KELLAWAY is a trans, queer, biracial writer, and the coeditor of *Manning Up*, an anthology of personal narratives by trans men. He covers transgender news for *Advocate.com* and has published with *Lambda Literary Review*, *Everyday Feminism*, *Huffington Post* and *Original Plumbing*. He is assistant editor for Transgress Press.

BELLE KNOX is an award-winning pornography actress and a feminist activist. She has contributed to *Time*, *Rolling Stone*, *Jezebel*, *XoJane*, *Huffington Post* and *Forbes* on the topics of feminism, sexual freedom, censorship and libertarianism. A women's studies student at Duke University and a Students for Liberty Campus Coordinator, Belle has spoken at Duke University, UNC Chapel Hill, Lafayette College and the International Conference on Human Trafficking.

JIZ LEE (JizLee.com) is a queer porn star whose video work spans a decade of more than two hundred projects over three continents. The genderqueer performer is founder of the erotic philanthropic Karma Pervs, and editor of the porn anthology *How to Come Out Like a Porn Star*.

ASHLEY MANTA (AshleyManta.com) is a feminist sexuality educator and writer and author of the e-book, *A Feminist's Guide to Phone Sex* (Frisky Feminist Press, 2014). Ashley speaks candidly about living with herpes and has done extensive work to promote acceptance and break the stigma surrounding STIs. She is cohost of sex and relationship podcast Carnalcopia.

CAMERYN MOORE (camerynmoore.com) is a playwright/performer, free-range writer, accidental educator, and yes, a phone sex operator. Her first play *Phone Whore* won the award for Best Female Solo show at the 2010 San Francisco Fringe Festival and Critics' Choice at the 2013 Houston Fringe Festival.

JARRETT NEAL earned a BA in English from Northwestern University and an MFA in Writing from the School of the Art Institute of Chicago. His work has been featured in many publications, both online and in print, including *Cold Drank, The Gay and Lesbian Review, Chelsea Station, Q Review, Requited Journal* and *Off the Rocks.*

NICA NOELLE is a writer, director and producer of adult films who has created eight studios in the last decade, including Sweetheart Video, Sweet Sinner Films, TransRomantic, Girl Candy Films and gay romance line Icon Male. Her writing regularly appears in The Huffington Post, Salon.com and a variety of other print magazines and newspapers.

CHARLIE NOX is a (semiretired) dating coach, OKCupid expert and award-winning sex blogger. She specializes in working with people with significant barriers to dating and was voted one of the Top 100 Sex Bloggers of 2012 and one of the Top 100 Sex Blogging Superheroes of 2013.

MORGAN M. PAGE (Odofemi.com) is a transsexual performance and video artist, writer, blogger, activist and Santera in Montréal. In 2013, she was the recipient of two SF MOTHA awards (New/Upcoming Artist of the Year and Group Exhibition, TWAT/fest), and she is a 2014 Lambda Literary fellow. Her first novel is forthcoming from Topside Press.

JOAN PRICE (joanprice.com) is the author of *The Ultimate Guide to Sex After Fifty: How to Maintain—or Regain!—a Spicy, Satisfying Sex Life*; *Better Than I Ever Expected: Straight Talk about Sex After Sixty* and *Naked at Our Age: Talking Out Loud about Senior Sex*.

CORY SILVERBERG (sexuality.about.com) is a sexuality educator, author and trainer. He received his Masters of Education from the Ontario Institute for Studies in Education and trains across North America on topics including access and inclusion, sexuality and disability, and sex and technology.

DAVID HENRY STERRY (davidhenrysterry.com), author of sixteen books, is a performer and activist. His bestselling memoir *Chicken Self: Portrait of a Man for Rent* has been translated into a dozen languages. *Hos, Hookers, Call Girls and Rent Boys* was featured on the cover of the Sunday *New York Times Book Review*.

STOYA is an adult performer and writer. She recommends that you refrain from Googling her while at work. Read more of her words at graphicdescriptions.com.

EMBER SWIFT is a Canadian musician, songwriter, performer and writer currently based in Beijing who maintains three popular blogs through her website (emberswift.com). She is an opinion writer for China.org as well as a contributing writer for *Herizon's Magazine, Mami Magazine, Beijing Kids Magazine* (and online blog) and InCulture Parent, an online portal for cross-cultural parenting.

ALOK VAID-MENON (returnthegayze.com) is a trans/national artist and activist writing and rioting for racial and economic justice. They are currently on tour with DarkMatter, a trans South Asian poetry collaboration, and work with the Audre Lorde Project, a community organizing center for queer people of color.

MOLLENA WILLIAMS is a writer, actress, BDSM Educator and storyteller, author of *The Toybag Guide: Taboo Play* and coauthor of *Playing Well With Others: Your Guide to Discovering, Exploring and Navigating the Kink, Leather and BDSM Communities* with Lee Harrington. Her essays appear in several anthologies including Tristan Taormino's *The Ultimate Guide to Kinky Sex*.

CHRISTOPHER ZEISCHEGG spent eight years working in the adult film industry as performer Danny Wylde. He's been a contributor to *The Feminist Porn Book* and a variety of online publications, such as *Medium* and *Nerve*. His second novel, *The Wolves that Live in Skin and Space*, will be published in 2015 through Rare Bird Books.

About the Editor

JON PRESSICK (SexinWords.ca) is a Toronto-based writer, editor, blogger, radio personality and gadabout specializing in topics related to sex and sexuality for more than fifteen years. Currently, Jon contributes to Kinkly.com and has been published on/in *New York Magazine*, MetAnotherFrog.com, *Xtra*, *Quill & Quire* and in the books *Secrets of the Sex Masters* and *Best Sex Writing 2013*. He primarily publishes to his blog, Sex in Words, sharing and contributing analysis of sex-related news stories, feature interviews and erotic fiction.

As one of the hosts and producer of Toronto's sex radio institution Sex City, Jon has interviewed some of the sex community's biggest names, including Cindy Gallop, Candida Royalle, Sunny Megatron, Susie Bright, Tristan Taormino, Kate McCombs, Reid Mihalko, Carol Queen, Dr. Charlie Glickman and many others (including many of the contributors to this collection).

When he pulls himself away from the keyboard, Jon occasionally performs burlesque, DJs, speaks at sexuality conferences, acts as a juror for the Feminist Porn Awards, curates an erotica library and offers prostate pleasure and erotica workshops.

Throughout the years, Jon's efforts have earned him TNT's Sex Journalist of the Year Award and recognition as one of Broken Pencil's "50 People and Places We Love."

Grateful acknowledgment is made for permission to reprint the following essays:

"Captain Save-A-Ho" was published in *Johns, Marks, Tricks and Chickenhawks: Professionals & Their Clients Writing about Each Other* (Soft Skull Press, 2013). "How a Former Porn Star's Sex Tape Helped Him Reclaim His Sex Life" by Christopher Zeischegg aka Danny Wylde was published April 3, 2014 on Nerve. "What Should We Call Sex Toys?" by Epiphora was published on February 8, 2013 on Hey Epiphora! "We Need A New Orientation to Sex" by Cory Silverberg was published October 16, 2013 on Huffington Post. "I Am the Blogger Who Allegedly 'Complicated' the Steubenville Rape Case" by Alexandria Goddard was published on March 18, 2013 on xojane.com. Reprinted with permission from xojane.com, http://www.xojane.com/issues/steubenville-rape-verdict-alexandria-goddard. "Porn Director: I Changed My Mind about Condoms" by Nica Noelle was published September 27, 2013 on Salon. "Pregger Libido" by Ember Swift was published September 25, 2013 on Ember Swift. "The White Kind of Body" by Alok Vaid-Menon was published on August 10, 2012 on Queer Libido. "Sex, Lies and Public Education" by Lynn Comella was published May 31, 2013 on Vegas Seven. "Sharing Body Heat" by Joan Price was published August 2, 2013 on Huffington Post. "Being a Real-Life Accomplice" by Cameryn Moore was published December 17, 2013 on Cameryn Moore. "Oops, I Slept With Your Boyfriend" by Charlie Nox was published August 26, 2013 on Huffington Post. "Pump Dreams" by Mitch Kellaway was published in *Cliterature: The Clitoris,* Vol. XXIX. "Prostitution Law and the Death of Whores" by Laura Agustín was published August 15, 2013 on Jacobin. "Fisting Day" by Jiz Lee was published in *The Feminist Porn Book* edited by Tristan Taormino, Constance Penley, Celine Parrenas Shimisu and Mireille Miller-Young (The Feminist Press, 2013). "Tell Me You Want Me." by Mollena Williams was published July 4, 2013 on The Perverted Negress. "The Gates" by Tina Horn was originally published in the MFA thesis "Useful Notes on the Modern Sex Worker," (Sarah Lawrence College, May 2013). "The Choice of Motherhood and Insidious Drugstore Signage" by Stoya was published May 12, 2013 on Stoya.tumblr.com. "Kinky, Sober and Free: BDSM in Recovery" was published April 17, 2013 on The Fix. "Crazy Trans Woman Syndrome" by Morgan M. Page was published January 17, 2013 on Odofemi. "Let's Talk about Interracial Porn" by Jarrett Neal was published in *The Gay and Lesbian Review,* July/August 2013. "When I Was a Birthday Present for an Eighty-Two-Year-Old Grandmother" by David Henry Sterry was published in *Chicken: Self-Portrait of a Young Man for Rent* (Soft Skull Press, 2013). "What an Armpit Model Taught Me About Sexual Language" by Jon Pressick was published January 28, 2014 on Sex in Words. "Growing Through the Yuck" by Ashley Manta was published April 18, 2013 on Herpes Life. "I Was A Teenage Porn Model" by Lux Alptraum was published October 15, 2013 on Medium. "Disability and Sex" by Jason Armstrong was published August 3, 2013 on Hunting for Sex: Cautionary Tales from the Quest. "Fumbling Towards Humanity: How 'Trans Grrrls' Helped Me Open Up to My Partner" by Amy Dentata was published April 21, 2014 on Pink Label. "In Defense of Celibacy" by Lauren Marie Fleming, aka Queerie Bradshaw was published April 5, 2013 on Queerie Bradshaw. "No Restrictions" by Dee Dee Behind was published in *Prose and Lore,* Issue 2.